MOLECULAR GODS

BOOKS BY PHILIP B. APPLEWHITE

Organizational Behavior

*Studies in Organizational Behavior and
Management, Second Edition*
(with Donald E. Porter and Michael J. Misshauk)

Focus: Biology

Understanding Biology (with Sam Wilson)

Philip B. Applewhite

MOLECULAR GODS

How Molecules Determine Our Behavior

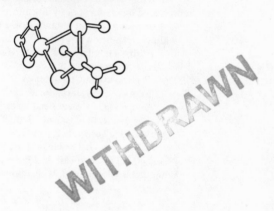

PRENTICE-HALL, INC.,
Englewood Cliffs, New Jersey

Lines from "voices to voices, lip to lip" by E.E.
Cummings are reprinted from *Is 5*, by E.E. Cummings,
with permission of Liveright Publishing Corporation,
Copyright 1926 by Horace Liveright, copyright
renewed 1954 by E.E. Cummings.

Illustrations by Linda Price Thomson

Art Director: Hal Siegel
Book Designer: Linda Huber

Library of Congress Cataloging in Publication Data

Applewhite Philip B
Molecular gods.
Includes index.
1. Psychology, Physiological.
2. Orthomolecular psychiatry. I. Title.
QP360.A66   152   80-22834
ISBN 0-13-599530-2

*To Harriet, who is beginning to believe
in molecular gods;
to Ellie, Katie, and Dougie,
who still are not sure;
and to Madame Max Goesler and Phineas Finn,
who could not care less.*

Acknowledgments

I thank my typist, Lorraine A. Klump, for her superb job of manuscript preparation and continually cheerful comments. I gratefully acknowledge the reading of my manuscript at various stages of preparation by Peter Levy, Robert Satter, Ruth Satter, Edith Poor, and Joseph Reagan. They corrected errors of fact, pointed out omissions, and suggested what needed reworking. Darline Levy kept me up for this book for two years while contributing her enthusiasm, her energy, and above all her unlimited intelligence. My wife, Harriet, has shared twenty years of her thinking with me, and it has profoundly affected all my writing, while delaying her own.

Preface

We all wonder why we do some of the things we do, and this book attempts to explain why. My purpose in writing is to inform the general public about behavior in a brief introduction to a complex problem, but I will show how molecules determine our behavior, and demonstrate that there can be no behavior without molecules being involved. The molecular study of behavior is a relatively young field, so it is not possible to give the final explanation of each and every behavior. My explanations are sometimes no more than guesses about what may be happening within us; they are certainly not the only molecular explanations possible. Nevertheless, they are based on available scientific facts. The explanations I offer are bound to be modified as research continues, but the molecular nature of behavior will be confirmed, extended, and established as the explanation of choice. It will change the way we look at ourselves.

Contents

MOLECULAR GODS

1

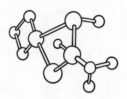

Molecular Gods at Work

Our behavior is controlled by molecules—by nothing else. Every thought, every movement, and every gesture of ours depends upon the right molecule being at the right place at the right time in our bodies. A molecule is made up of two or more atoms held together by physical forces, and we, like everything else, are made of molecules. While they shape our noses and mold our feet, they also cause us to be aggressive or passive, fat or thin, creative or dull, homosexual or heterosexual, mentally ill or happy. These molecules act as gods, so to speak, ruling us perhaps more than we imagine. If this is the case, then our behavior owes more to the molecular events within us than to the events around us.

Behavior is what we do with ourselves. It encompasses everything we do, whether it is daydreaming, making decisions about our life, or just having fun.

Because our molecules determine our behavior, we may have no control over how we behave in some cases, and could even use this fact to excuse our behavior. What is better than to call our selfishness, aggressiveness, materialism, and hatefulness a molecular and not a personal problem? If our molecules are to blame, then we can curse them first and not the people and the society around us.

Make no mistake about it, when we engage in a behavior we make our molecules move around. But since we are merely a collection of molecules ourselves, there is no "we" apart from molecules. Our behavior consists of some molecules moving other molecules around. There is not a group of molecules that is "us" and another group of molecules that is not us. It is therefore incorrect to say that we control our molecules or that our molecules control us, because that implies there is a "we" not made of molecules —and there is not. To be precise, when I say our molecules control us in ways that we do not expect or in ways that we do not like, I mean that some of the molecules in our body are not under the control of other molecules that should control them.

PSYCHOLOGICAL VERSUS MOLECULAR EXPLANATIONS OF BEHAVIOR Once we acknowledge our molecular nature, we can easily see that there is a molecular alternative to the psychological explanations of behavior we are so familiar with. Psychologists attempt to explain our behavior by looking at the influences other people, places, things, and events (the environment) have had on us. They would argue that one becomes a schizophrenic, a loving person, or an alcoholic because of

2

one's personal experiences in life. I will argue that we are what we are because of what our molecules are doing. What we become may well be influenced by the people, places, things, and events around us—but only if they affect our molecules. Furthermore, we shall see that molecules move and change in our bodies and determine some behaviors totally independently of what happens around us. We do not always have to attribute a present behavior to past experiences.

Typically we say that people who act strangely—whether they be public figures, artists, or the mentally ill—are merely responding to past psychological experiences that have somehow shaped their lives and their work. It may be that they are not responding to past life-events but rather to surprising molecular changes within their brains that have occurred independently of what passed around them. While these people—and in fact all of us—may have had quite eventful experiences in growing up, it becomes impossible to prove the relevance of these experiences to any given subsequent behavior. We do not and cannot know how we would behave if we lived our lives differently, and if we were exposed to different experiences.

WHAT REALLY CAUSES OUR BEHAVIOR? We generally assume that if our parents had been different, or if they interacted differently with us, or if we were raised in another part of the country, or if life were better to us, we would be different in our behavior. But we can never know if this is in fact true. There are, of course, many studies that have demonstrated if one group of people are treated one way, and another group treated another way, there will be differences in behavior between the groups. For example, if one group of factory or office workers is lectured to and told to do their job differently, they will resist this change more than another identical group given the information more gently and then allowed to discuss it with management. You can also take a nice dog and train it to attack anyone it does not know. The environment is clearly at work here. But in the absence of such studies, an explanation of any given person's behavior that is based on his or her past personal history is just speculation.

To prove that one event causes another to occur, we have to subject two identical people or things to two different conditions. One person is subjected only to the event and the other one is not. If one person changes and the other does not, then we can say that the event caused something to happen. For example, does light cause plants to grow? We look and we see all sorts of things that might affect growth besides light: temperature, humidity, water, wind, and soil conditions. The only way to determine if light causes plants to grow is to subject one plant to light and another identical plant to no light (i.e., dark) while keeping all the other conditions (like temperature, etc.) the same for both plants. If the plants are not identical to start with, the initial differences between them may account for the final differences also. For instance, if the plant put in the dark is much older to begin with, it might not grow much even if it were in the light. We would not know then whether light causes the plant in the light to grow or whether old age causes the plant in the dark not to grow. If this experiment is performed properly, we will see that the plant in the light grows more than the one in the dark. Since the only difference between the plants is the presence of light, we can say that light caused the growth.

It is far more difficult to prove causation with human behavior. First of all, where do we obtain identical people to subject to different conditions? Identical twins are the only possibility. They result from the fusion of only one sperm with only one egg. The fertilized egg soon divides into two embryos rather than producing just one embryo. Identical twins are as close together as they can be genetically since they have arisen from the same egg genes and sperm genes. On the other hand, fraternal twins develop from separate eggs and separate sperm. They are genetically no more similar than siblings born years apart (to the same mother and father). One's siblings, after all, have developed from another egg and another sperm. Each egg from the same mother carries somewhat different genes, as does each sperm from the same father—that is why we look different from our nonidentical-twin brothers and sisters.

In the plant experiment mentioned above, obtaining identical plants is easy. We can take two cells from a plant leaf and in the laboratory nourish each cell into a complete plant. This is called cloning. For humans, we cannot send in the clones so easily. We have to take the identical twins that are born—we cannot create them at will. To get at the causes of human behavior, we have to subject one of the identical twins to an environmental influence the other does not receive. We could certainly have one twin brush with a fluoride toothpaste and another brush with brand X, but who cares? The really interesting environmental influences on behavior such as stress, parental influence, social conditions, and the like cannot ethically be imposed upon humans as part of an experiment. We cannot yank one twin away from another at birth for the purpose of conducting research.

We will see in subsequent chapters, however, that occasionally identical twins do get separated soon after birth because the parents have died or were unable financially or emotionally to take care of them. Sometimes the twins can be tracked down and the different environments they were raised in looked at to try to determine what effect, if any, the environment had on the twins' behavior. But even in this ideal research situation we cannot assume (with the complex lives humans lead) that there will be only slight differences between the two social environments the twins live in. They will have different friends, parents, situations, and separate locations in space that are all confounded with each other. It becomes impossible (without unethically controlling the identical twins' lives) to sort out just what in their social environment influences their subsequent behavior to the same extent one can sort out the effect of light on plant growth.

Therefore, to say that one specific aspect of the environment causes a subsequent behavior in any given person is not often possible because we do not have enough experimental control over the people or the environment to determine just what causes what. Send people to prison, annoy them, or take away their possessions and watch them change their behavior. The environment changes and their behavior changes. Fine—there is no argument. But the important question is: What influence upon subsequent behavior will these situations have when they have long since passed? It is the answer to this question that I am arguing is so difficult to answer, even using identical twins.

It is also possible that environmental factors may have no effect on some behaviors. Some random gathering of molecules in the brain, acting independently of the environment, may be the responsible force for many of our behaviors. To be sure, this is just as difficult to prove as an environmental influence, but it is no less valid an explanation. When one sees the macabre fantasies of such painters as René Magritte and Salvador Dali, for example, or reads the psychological novels of a James Joyce or Marcel Proust, or looks at the abhorrent acts of a Jack the Ripper or Joseph Stalin, it is tempting to offer explanations of their strange work or deviant behavior based on unique experiences they must have had in their lives. These men are certainly unique, but is the uniqueness drawn from their interaction with their social environment or from their molecules? We must not always assume the environment explains all. How can we be sure that a stressful infancy, a bad childhood, a traumatic adolescence or an unhappy adulthood shaped these men?

THE ROLE OF RANDOMNESS   There is no doubt that the environment within which we are embedded can influence our behavior. The death of a person we love makes us sad and the birth of a healthy baby makes us happy. But these events, as we shall see, utilize molecules and move them around in our brain to produce our feelings of sadness or happiness. These same feelings may spring up within us for no apparent reason. We can point to nothing in particular causing them, but molecules are still the culprit. We can have no feelings without molecules being involved; we can have no behavior without molecules being involved. If molecular changes arise randomly and then persist within our body, then it becomes possible to suggest that a wide variety of behaviors would develop independently of what the environment does to us. This is of great significance because it means that we cannot always help what we are.

We do not give randomness enough credit in our affairs. If you do not believe this, ask yourself why you are not starving in Cambodia or Laos or an innocent victim of any airplane hijacking, or a person caught in the weapons crossfire of a revolution. Our individuality, in fact, stems from randomness. A random sperm fertilizes a random egg which develops into a fetus born, as far as you are concerned, in a random place in the world. Our parents chose each other, but had no control over which sperm fertilized which egg. Even for test-tube babies, the sperm and egg used are chosen on the basis of which ones look healthy. They are not chosen on the basis of what molecules lurk within. While our genes direct our development from fertilization onward to maturity, there are plenty of opportunities for random events to affect our subsequent behavior.

If an event is random, it is unpredictable, because the event has the same chance of occurring in anyone. In everyday conversation we often use the word *random* to cover up our ignorance of the real cause of something. For example, cancer was thought to strike people at random. But as we learned more about the disease, it became apparent that people exposed to excessive amounts of radiation or certain chemicals were likely to get cancer. We could predict. Some behaviors may be influenced by truly random events because by chance some molecules in our brain end up at the wrong place at the wrong time. On the other hand, as we learn more about the molecular basis of behavior we may find that some seemingly random behaviors are not random at all, and that we can predict what is going to happen to whom.

INTERNAL VERSUS EXTERNAL CAUSES OF BE-HAVIOR Our sense of balance, sense of motion, and sense of limb position receive information from inside our body as to what is happening. Our senses of vision, touch, hearing, taste, and smell, on the other hand, receive information from outside the body. If any psychological (involving another person) or sociological (involving groups of people) event around us is to affect us, it can only do so through these senses. If we cannot see it, touch it, hear it, taste it, or smell it, it will not get into our brain. If it does not get in, it cannot have any effect upon our behavior. The function of these senses is to bring all kinds of information into our brain to allow us to react to the environment. These senses immediately translate the environment into molecular messages within our nervous system. While this occurs very quickly, it still takes a measurable amount of time, so by the time we have sensed something, it is past. Without being too philosophical about this we can say that there is therefore no present, only a past. Nor is there a future until we experience it, at which time it becomes the past.

Once what is happening in the environment is converted into molecular activities by our senses, it is no longer a psychological or sociological phenomenon involving people, places, things, and events. It is now molecular. Events external to the body have been transformed into internal bodily events. We may react immediately to this information or it may be stored in memory to be acted on later. Our reactions are called behavior and are expressed in two broad categories as either thinking or movement. We think about the stimuli we are continuously receiving, or we move and act in response to them. There are no other possibilities. Movement is not as limited a behavior as it might seem, since talking involves jaw and tongue movements, facial expressions involve movement of face muscles, and body gestures—such as aggressive actions—require limb movement. The mentally ill, champion athletes, homosexuals, the happy and the sad, the obese, the learning disabled, and all the rest can be characterized by how they think (what's going on in their brains) and how they move.

Behavior is anything a person does, whether the stimulus for it originates internally or externally or both. Hunger is an example of how both sources affect behavior. At mealtime our biological rhythms are such that molecular changes within the stomach produce nervous-system sensations of hunger in the brain—with no food in sight. But the sight and smell of food can also produce these feelings of hunger. Our behavior is then to want to eat, accomplished by the movement of arm, hand, and finger muscles to bring food to the mouth, followed by the lip, tongue, and jaw movements of chewing. Eating is a lot more fun than this, thank goodness. Nevertheless hunger offers a clear case of external and internal events working together to produce behavior, and either one of the events would be sufficient to cause hunger. Both are molecular changes that produce further molecular changes in us.

What we wish to determine is whether other kinds of more complex behaviors we exhibit can also be generated by molecules within us, independently of external events. If so, then those behaviors that make up our personalities may not be so easily explained by psychological theories that rely on people, places, things, and events external to us as the ultimate cause of behavior.

MIND-BODY PROBLEMS   It is not a question of whether molecules or psychological or sociological factors produce behavior, because psychological and sociological events entering the senses must produce molecular changes before they can affect behavior. This fact is not generally acknowledged in our everyday conversations, where we continually make distinctions between psychological and physical or biological causes. If we see people acting not themselves and see no obvious physical problem, we say they have a psychological problem. His or her mind has been affected in some way by disturbing interactions with other people, places, things, or events. The distinction is often made quite clearly between the physical and psychological. In reality, there is no such distinction, since psychological information must come into our brain through our senses, where it is physically transformed into molecular events. The ultimate cause of behavior can only be molecular.

The separation of ourselves into those parts that have a psychological basis and those that have a physical basis has been called the mind-body problem. There is no problem, however. The mind is the brain, the brain is part of the body, and the body is an assembly of molecules. There is no evidence whatsoever that there is a part of the brain called the mind. The "mind" has just been a convenient box in which to throw all the mysteries of the brain—and there are many mysteries. Unfortunately, the mysteries have taken on a form all their own, and have been considered by some to be the driving force within or apart from the brain. The mind in the brain is "the ghost in the machine." History has seen many such ghosts lose their white sheets—this one should be no different. We have lost the ghosts that pushed the planets around, the ghosts that made the winds blow, and the ghosts that caused disease. "From ghoulies and ghosties and long-leggety beasties . . . Good Lord, deliver us!"

Can molecules explain everything about ourselves? Can we measure how beautiful spring* is or how much love there is in a roomful of friends by weighing molecules or tracking their movements? Of course we cannot; we might not even want to. But we cannot say it will be impossible to do so in the future. Most of what we can do now was never even imagined: heart transplants,

---

*"while you and I have lips and voices which/are for kissing and to sing with/who cares if some one-eyed son of a bitch/invents an instrument to measure spring with?" e.e. cummings

brain-wave analysis, genetic engineering, and moving faster than the speed of sound. The future will always be different from the present.

CHEMICALS IN YOUR FUTURE Because of their molecular nature, all behaviors can in principle be treated (augmented or diminished) chemically. Whether we suffer from unrequited love, feelings of guilt, or alcoholism, there is a chemical in our future to help. As new drugs are developed, they are used; they do not just sit on the chemist's shelf. Similarly, as long as scientists are allowed to study behavior, more and more body chemicals will be implicated; drugs will be developed to interact with them in attempts to modify behavior.

Chemical behavior modification started slowly, like most other scientific endeavors. The aims were modest. Why not chemically control a body tremor, why not develop sleeping pills to help insomniacs or amphetamines to help those fatigued? These drugs are abused, but their ability to modify behavior in many people is not questioned. Did anyone ask you about this? Will anyone ask you whether it is all right to develop drugs to inhibit memory loss or to make you happier? New applications of drugs to modify behavior slip right in and we hardly notice them. Chemical modification of behavior grows year by year. It becomes more serious as it comes closer to changing our personality in more permanent ways. Behavior changes of this sort will also threaten those in power, because we will not have to rely on them for our happiness and sense of well-being if a pill or drug will do it.

Where does one draw the line and say, "No more research in this area because it is dangerous"? Guidelines may be developed and laws even passed. This has been done for the so-called recombinant DNA experiments where functioning human genes have been introduced into bacteria and recombined with their genes. The fear has been that we will get our genes mixed up.

It is very difficult to stop the acquisition of knowledge because people keep thinking, and passing the knowledge to others, and once the knowledge is acquired it is impossible to get rid of all memories of it. We cannot now stop people from designing nuclear weapons, supersonic aircraft, or large automobiles, because the facts for their creation are available. But we can make it difficult for people actually to build them. We begin to make it difficult when we realize we may be worse off with the product, but there is really no way to stop the acquisition of new knowledge.

When we realize we have the potential to change our behavior in a very fundamental way—with the molecules where it develops—we will have a momentous decision to make. Should we do it, or should we accept ourselves as we are and do all we can to modify the social conditions around us to get the best of what our unaltered molecules can give us? When we see how much we can change our behavior by molecular intervention, we may prefer to use the social methods we have at our disposal and change our environment. We could make serious efforts to get rid of racial and religious prejudice, unemployment, poverty, and bad nutrition and starvation. We

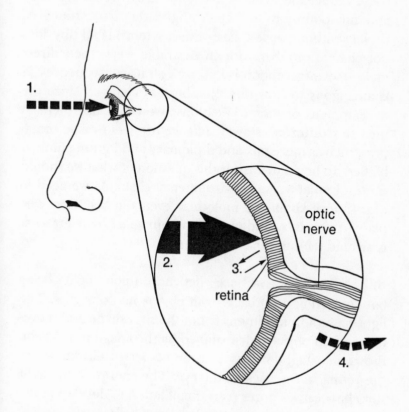

Figure 1: **MOLECULAR CHANGES FROM SEEING**
Light is reflected from the environment (1) into the eye (2).
The light strikes the cells of the retina within the eye (3).
Molecules and atoms move in and out of these cells. Nerve
impulses are created and move along the optic nerve (4) to the
brain where they are interpreted.

could reduce the stress of living in cities by reducing noise and air pollution; we could fight the frustrations of driving with improved mass-transit sytems. If all this does not change our behavior in desirable ways, then direct molecular intervention is left, with all its consequences. It is analogous to how our thinking has changed since the development of atomic weapons. We could use them to melt our differences away, but we use less drastic measures, such as more talk and diplomacy and fighting limited battles. To begin to answer this question of what we should do (molecular versus environmental change), we need to know more about the molecular events in behavior. The place to start is by finding out how our senses convert what is around us into molecular events.

SEEING What we see depends upon light being bounced (reflected) back from objects into our eyes. The light has color and intensity but the size, shape and movement of an object is determined by the image it makes on the retina. Light strikes a group of nerve cells known as the retina in the back of the eye. The energy of the light somehow causes pores (very small holes) to develop in the membranes that surround the nerve cells in the retina, thereby allowing some molecules and atoms (the building blocks of molecules) to move in and others to move out of these cells.

These molecular and atomic movements generate nerve impulses, which travel to the brain via optic nerves for interpretation of what we see ("the eye sees not of itself but by reflection"). Nerve impulses are transmitted from one part of the body to another along nerves in much the same way as a stack of dominoes falls. Molecular changes at one location in a nerve cause molecular changes to take place right next to that location, and so on down the nerve. In keeping with the domino analogy, the dominoes would have to be set up again, because the molecular changes at any one spot on the nerve last only a few thousandths of a second in order to give the nerve a chance to transmit another message if necessary.

The molecular movements produced in the nerve cells of the eye are not random, but are coded in a nerve-impulse language to represent what we see. If any visual event is to affect our behavior, it must first be converted into these molecular changes in the eye (Figure 1 illustrates the events occurring in vision). Conversely, molecular events in the eye can affect how we see. It is known, for example, that at the time of ovulation, human females can see better in the dark than at other times in the menstrual cycle. This may be due to certain increased hormonal levels in the blood at this time that increase the ease with which molecules and atoms move through the cellular pores. Could it be that this trait was useful when we lived in caves tens of thousands of years ago to help find a mate in the dark? Some think so.

HEARING Sound waves, like light waves, are also converted into molecular changes. Sounds are waves in the air (like ripples on the surface of water) and are characterized by their intensity and frequency. Frequency refers to the number of times per second the sound waves strike our eardrums. At our peak (which you have probably

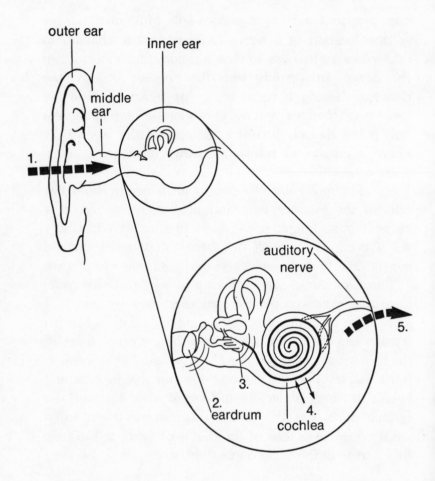

Figure 2: MOLECULAR CHANGES FROM HEARING
Sound waves enter the ear (1) and vibrate the eardrum (2) which moves the tiny bones of the ear (3). Their movements produce molecular changes in the cochlea (4) that lead to nerve impulses being transmitted to the brain (5).

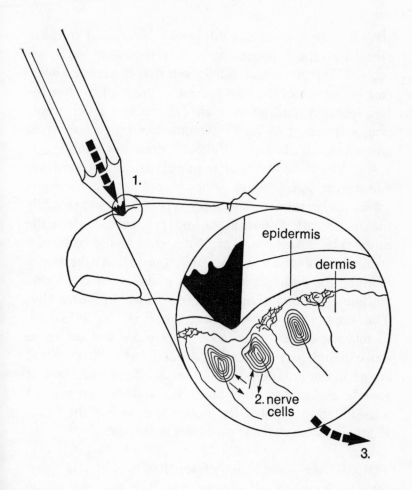

Figure 3: **MOLECULAR CHANGES FROM TOUCHING**
When the skin is touched (1), nerve cells in it are slightly
squashed (2). This causes molecular changes in them, and
the production of nerve impulses for the brain (3).

passed if you are reading this book) we can hear frequencies from about sixteen to twenty thousand waves per second. Expensive high-fidelity sets that produce frequencies greater than this are wasted on most of us, but the frequencies sound good in advertisements. When someone is speaking to us, the frequencies range only from about a hundred to three thousand times per second.

When the waves strike our eardrums, the eardrum vibrates at a frequency proportional to the incoming waves, and in turn vibrates three very small bones (actually the three smallest bones in the body) connected to it on the inner side. These bones are connected to the cochlea, a small fluid-filled sac deep within the ear. As the bones vibrate, the fluid in the cochlea also vibrates. These vibrations are picked up by nerve cells within the cochlea. The energy of the vibrations changes the nerve-cell membrane structure to allow molecules and atoms to move in and out of pores, just as occurred in the retina, to create nerve impulses. The molecular representations of sounds are sent to the brain via auditory nerves for interpretation of what the noises are outside the body. Figure 2 indicates these processes in the ear.

TOUCHING Our sense of touch also depends upon changes in nerve-cell membranes. The pressure of an object on our skin ever so slightly deforms the membranes of nerve cells scattered along our skin and causes, just as with vision and hearing, molecules and atoms to move across the nerve-cell membranes. This produces nerve impulses which first are sent to the spinal cord and then to the brain. The nerve impulses have coded within them just how hard we have been touched; their location indicates where we were touched. Was it a kiss or did we get belted? We need to know how to respond. Located within the skin are other nerve cells which respond to heat, cold, and pain in much the same way as the touch-sensitive nerve cells do. Figure 3 illustrates touch sensations.

SMELLING AND TASTING   Our senses of smell and taste, also represented by molecular changes, depend not on physical modes of stimulation like light, sound, and the pressure of touch, but on molecules themselves. In order for us to smell or taste something, molecules must be given off by the object. Everything is made up of atoms, and there are only ninety-two kinds of atoms that occur in nature on earth. Some familiar kinds of atoms are oxygen, neon, calcium, iron, iodine, aluminum, silver, and gold. Atoms are usually bound together to form molecules. When hydrogen and oxygen bind together we get water; with sodium and chloride we get table salt. To get a living thing we need more kinds of atoms, but only about twenty of the ninety-two types available. Together, atoms and molecules are the building blocks of all substances, whether it be a brain, a drain, a chair, or air. It is remarkable how only ninety-two types of atoms have combined into molecules to produce everything in this world—and out of it, as far as we know.

When food (or any other substance) is in our mouth, some of its molecules fall off or are loosened by our saliva and lodge in our taste buds, located in the tongue. There the molecules fit into any of thousands of different recesses in the nerve-cell membranes of the taste buds. A force between these food molecules and molecules in the membranes is developed that opens pores in the membranes, allowing molecules and atoms to move in and out of the nerve cells to produce nerve impulses.

We smell things in much the same way, except here, the molecules of an object come loose before they reach the nose. A few molecules bounce loose from just about everything, but those that lose the most, smell the most—people included. Once in the nose, they also land in recesses in membranes of nerve cells, with the resultant production of nerve impulses representing the smell. The molecules entering the mouth or nose carry with them, as part of their molecular structure, information about taste or smell which the nervous system responds to. If a substance does not give off molecules, it will have no taste or smell. Figures 4 and 5 illustrate these processes. Whatever sense it is, it transforms external information into internal information.

EXTRASENSORY PERCEPTION   Even if you believe in ESP (extra sensory perception), the signals coming in from another person must still be picked up by some nerve cells and converted to molecular events and nerve impulses before we can be aware of the signals. The term extrasensory perception implies a signal is detected by something other than our five senses. This does not have to be a totally mysterious event, for all one has to do to bring these events within the realm of contemporary science is to suggest that we have, as yet, an undetected sense (complete with nerve cells, membranes, and associated molecules) waiting to be found. Many animals (such as migrating birds) alter their flying behavior in response to the earth's magnetic field. Tying a small magnet around such a bird will disrupt its navigational abilities for a while. Scientists do not know what special sense is involved, but there certainly is one.

INDIVIDUAL AND GROUP BEHAVIOR   If molecules are responsible for individual behavior, then they are also responsible for group behavior. It is often said that a group is more than just the sum of its individuals. We can observe that an angry mob is more frightening than just a lot of angry individuals, and a government is more complicated than just a lot of people doing their individual jobs. It is the social interaction between people that makes a group different from its component individuals. However, social interactions like all other influences can have an effect upon us only after being converted into molecular events by our senses. Therefore I would claim that we could understand the behavior of any group—be it the United Nations, a country, a company, or a group of friends—by studying the molecules of the individuals involved. A fuller discussion of group behavior goes beyond the scope of this book (which means I do not wish to write about it anymore), but it is important to realize just what a molecular approach can accomplish.

MOLECULAR THEOLOGY   If our life is so dominated by molecules, how did we get this way? We did not vote on it; we were made this way. The earth is about five billion years old, and living things are thought to have been around for the last three billion years or so. Evolutionary

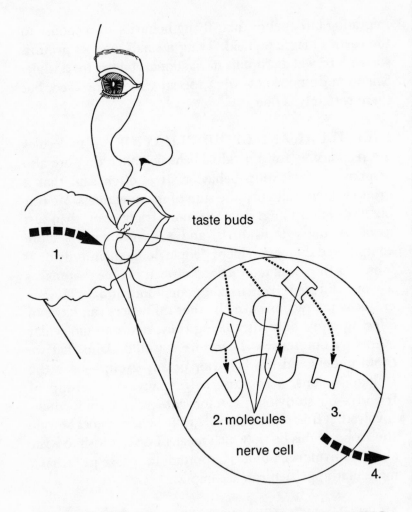

taste buds

1.

2. molecules

3.

nerve cell

4.

Figure 4: **MOLECULAR CHANGES FROM TASTING**
Objects that have a taste (1) give off molecules (2) in the
mouth, where they attach to cells in our taste buds (3).
Molecular changes are produced by these attachments and are
transmitted as nerve impulses (4) to the brain.

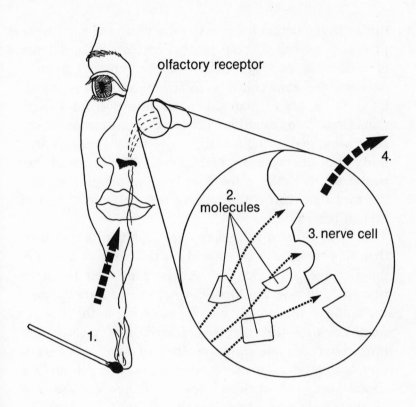

olfactory receptor

2.
molecules

3. nerve cell

4.

1.

Figure 5: **MOLECULAR CHANGES FROM SMELLING**
*Objects that have an odor (1) give off molecules (2) that enter
the nose, where they attach to certain nerve cells (3). Molecular
changes in the nerve cells produce the nerve impulses (4) that go
to the brain.*

theory suggests that the first organisms on the earth were primitive one-celled creatures that developed from a mix of chemicals and gradually became more chemically complex and multicelled as their environment changed. Of the diversity of plants, animals, and microorganisms that have arisen from these primitive organisms, some are still unchanged (living fossils), some have died off (extinction), and others have evolved into higher forms of life, where we modestly place ourselves—although someone has said that man is the missing link between apes and human beings.

An alternative to accepting evolution is to believe that all organisms were placed on the earth at different times. Some have died off, and we find their fossilized remains, but one life form did not evolve into another, according to this notion. No one was there at the time, so we do not know who, if anyone, placed them on earth; and no one has seen one animal evolve into another one—not even with a government research grant. There is endless speculation. God, working under a number of aliases, is a possibility. As one astronomer has suggested, spaceships may have visited us billions of years ago and dumped their sewage and garbage on earth. What they left chemically evolved into us. We may have every reason to feel like shit once in a while.

Another suggestion has been that organisms were placed here as an experiment by life forms far superior to ours. It makes no sense to estimate the probability of such a superior life form (or life of any sort) occurring in outer space. Either it does exist or it does not. We could be a zoological and botanical garden for it to observe, but we are no more aware of our keeper than the bacteria in our mouth are of theirs. Compared to ourselves, bacteria have no intelligence because we are billions of years more evolved. In turn, we would look pretty stupid to someone who is billions of years more evolved than we. So much so, perhaps, that they have lost interest in us and we have to fend for ourselves now. The universe may be twenty billion years old; as such, there would be fifteen billion more years than earth has had to work with in perfecting intelligence. It is rather sobering to consider that our wars, economic crises, food and energy shortages might be the manipulations of superior beings (experimenters) who wish to observe our behavior in a laboratory setting.

There is no solid evidence to tell us exactly how we became as we are, and there can never be any if we in fact evolved from simpler organisms than ourselves. The past can never be reconstructed in its totality. The fact that we cannot eliminate from our thinking the possibility that others have created us, or are controlling us, shows how little we really know about ourselves. Nevertheless, both religion and science claim to have the answers. The religious viewpoint offers its sacred texts as evidence for its point of view, while the scientific viewpoint offers its data, millions of years after the fact. Both explanations have their built-in assumptions which prevent us from objectively choosing one from another. Religions assume their texts are divinely inspired. Science assumes that given plenty of time, complex life forms arise from the simple. While this is demonstrably true of bureaucracies, it is impossible to prove for living things.

Regardless of which of the three most discussed possibilities for the origin of life on earth you prefer (evolution, God, experimenters), the fact remains that we are still constructed of molecules. Astronomers have found that many of the kinds of molecules found here on earth are also found in outer space, so we appear to have a supply of the necessary molecules. Those molecules were assembled from atoms, but where did the atoms come from? We assume something cannot come from nothing. Did God make them; did atoms always exist? We can only guess at the answers. According to evolutionary theory, two billion years was presumably enough time for atoms and molecules to combine randomly into a one-celled molecular package that remained relatively stable, was protected from the environment, could use energy from the sun, and could reproduce. This package we call Life. A central issue to us is whether the molecules were assembled into life randomly, or whether their assembly was directed. We get back to God or experimenters again as the directed assemblers, or evolution and the laws of nature as the random assemblers.

Since we are assembled of molecules, only those things that affect molecular structure or molecular location can have any effect upon us. This is exactly the way in which our senses operate. They affect us by affecting our molecules. The ultimate explanation of behavior must then come from an understanding of our molecules.

MOLECULAR REALITY Because we are made of molecules, all our actions must be produced by molecules. This does not diminish our worth or make us any less human. On the contrary, to deny our molecular makeup is to ignore our reality. Practically speaking, something is real if most people agree it exists. This definition of reality is, however, limited by our own ignorance. At one time reality consisted of thinking the earth was flat, because everyone believed it to be so. So what is real is not limited to what we think is real. Reality exists whether anyone observes it or not. Reality is limited ultimately only by the laws of physics that govern what molecules and atoms do. Unlike man-made laws, natural laws cannot be cast aside. If we wish to stop the world and get off, the laws of physics will allow us to do this only if we can obtain a speed of about twenty-four thousand miles per hour to escape the earth's gravity. There is no other way we can get off. We cannot fly without the aid of a machine, nor reproduce by hatching eggs—but not because of limits set by the laws of physics. After all, birds do these things and they do not violate any such laws. Rather, these limitations occur because we do not have the right molecules in the right places. In other words, our bodies do not have the necessary molecular structure to allow us to fly or lay eggs. We must therefore add a further limitation to what living things can do—the proper molecular structure must be present. This is reflected at all levels in the organism, for the molecules determine what the cells will be like, and the cells determine what our body will look like and how it will function. This design of structural information is in the molecules of our genes, which direct what our body will be like and consequently what our limitations will be. Our behavior always reflects these limitations. Designer genes have been around a long time.

MOLECULES—SO WHAT? So what does it matter if our behavior is produced by molecules? Does it make any difference if we can be specific about what molecules produce what behavior? Or are we just as well off to talk of such presently vague but commonly accepted aspects of behavior as motivation, the psyche, ego, feelings, and personality? After all, if we think someone is an ass, that says just as much as saying he or she is a little short of molecule X. However, if we wish to enhance or eliminate wanted or unwanted behaviors, then it matters very much to realize that molecular events cause them. For then we can deal directly with molecules without having to rely on environmental changes which might not be converted into the proper chemical changes.

Take mental illness, for example. If we have a molecular and genetic predisposition for it that is aggravated by a "stressful" environment, then we can either change the environment or directly change the molecules involved. The environment is converted by the senses into molecular events anyhow, so why not directly change the molecules causing behavior? This avoids taking a chance that the proper molecular events will not be produced by the environmental changes. If it is not clear what specific stresses led to the illness, it will not be clear what stresses to avoid in finding a new environment for the mentally ill. Furthermore, if the people, places, things, and events in our environment really have no relationship to the behavior or only contributes partially, then changing the environment can have no or little effect upon that behavior. Subsequent chapters will show that this may be the case with certain aspects of mental illness as well as with alcoholism, obesity, aggression, thinking, love, homosexuality, happiness, and personality traits. Actually, we will see that the environment alone cannot explain all our behaviors, because our body chemistry is always involved also. Therefore, changing only the environment can never change all our internal molecular events. Changing the environment will always be less efficient than changing our internal molecules directly, because the molecules are always directly involved in behavior. It is certainly easier to blame the environment for our problems—it is something we can see and touch, unlike molecules, which seem too small to matter. If the environment is not that important to understanding every behavior, then we need a complete reassessment of the ways to solve our behavior-related problems.

Knowing what the molecules are doing in us will also give us a more fundamental understanding of behavior. This means we can explain behavior with fewer variables (determining factors). Often, the less we know about something, the more variables we need to explain it. This is because we do not know which are the most important and which are the least important factors. We really are trying to cover all our bets. For instance, we know that our behavior is influenced at one time or another by our genes, physiology, diet, chance, parental influence, people we interact with, physical disabilities caused by disease or injury, world events, and just about anything else. While this is true of our behaviors taken as a whole, no one behavior is influenced by each of these factors to the same extent, if at all. To handle all these variables together would be a formidable task. We would need a knowledge of economics, sociology, political science, and history to deal with the impact of world events upon our behavior. We would need to know nutrition to determine proper vitamin levels, probability theory to deal with chance effects, and chemistry to understand our genes and physiology. We would also need to know psychology to determine what the influence of people on us will be, and microbiology to determine what the diseases are that affect behavior.

Fortunately, these factors all have one thing in common—molecules. No factor can have an effect until it is transformed into molecular events. Once we realize this, we have a common currency to handle all the possible influences on behavior. No effect on our molecules, no effect on our behavior. We have become more fundamental in our thinking as we have reduced the number of variables to explain behaviors down to one: molecules.

MOLECULES AND PSYCHOHISTORY Much effort is spent in studying our past in attempts to understand our present—or to better our future. On one level we want to explain such large-scale collective events as wars, revolutions, and social and economic development. On another level we want to understand individuals who have had an influence on the way the world is, for better or for worse. We wish to know why they behaved as they did and what we might do to foster the development of the good and hinder the bad. Did Adolf Hitler's upbringing play an important role in his decisions to exterminate ten million people in Europe? Did Martin Luther King's experiences as a young person lead to his commitment to the Civil

Rights Movement in the United States? Why those people? Certainly others experienced similar social conditions and yet did not do what these two men did. Their underlying molecular structures had to be a factor.

For those who already are dead, a direct molecular examination of their brain would reveal nothing. When we die, the energy (extracted from food) that maintains our molecular structure is no longer available to hold things together, and we begin to crumble. The white blood cells that provided our immunological defenses die, enabling microorganisms to attack our structure further. With molecular information on the dead unattainable, we are left with an incomplete picture of how their behavior was influenced. We would not know just what aspects of their environment were translated into molecular events, so we could never be sure what influence their life experience had upon them. It is fun to guess about the psychology of people in history but it is only a guess.

Biographies of famous people are continually appearing, and their authors inevitably look to their subject's social environment as the determinant of their subject's personality. Movie stars and other entertainers are prime targets for this kind of thinking. Janis Joplin, Judy Garland, and Marilyn Monroe self-destructed, it is said, because of too many demands placed upon them by their fans and the entertainment industry. How do we know they would be survivors if they did something else for a living? We do not know. Most biographical explanations of behavior are fanciful and are merely following the long-current vogue of accepting the environment and ignoring the biological makeup of an individual in explaining behavior. Biographers can easily dig up information about a person's past, but not about someone's biological makeup. Without this information, though, explanations of behavior are necessarily incomplete and should be considered sheer speculation.

Historians and biographers can reconstruct to varying degrees what sort of an environment a person lived in, including information about family and social life and the state of the world at the time. Maybe an analysis of the environmental influences does explain in some cases why people behave as they do. Maybe not. To ascertain the influence of the environment, one has to know the relative contribution of the inputs into the senses. Not all aspects of our environment influence us equally, so how are we to know what is important and what is not? Without looking inside the person, at molecular events, we cannot be sure what aspects of the environment entered the nervous system. This is not something we can determine on our own through introspection, either, so autobiographies are not much help. We cannot always remember accurately what may have happened to us. We are lacking the controlled experiment. We cannot go back in time to what we think are important events in our life and eliminate them, and then see—for comparison—whether we would still be the same person and behave the same way. This is the only way to determine how important a particular aspect of our environment was to our subsequent behavior.

In this age of psychology, psychotherapy, psychoanalysis, and "psychobabble," we have been taught to explain important aspects of our behavior on the basis of past events and the influences of people, places and things. We are *not* talking about each and every little behavior—such as scratching our nose, walking down the street, or opening a door—as having a deeper psychological meaning. We are talking about major behavioral features of our personality. No one is going to claim that the environment has no effect whatever upon our behavior. No one should claim, however, that the environment can affect us without first being converted into molecular events by our senses. No one should deny either that important aspects of our behavior may be caused by molecular events acting independently of what is happening around us. The following chapters will present specific examples of our molecular gods at work.

2

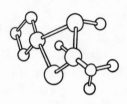

Biological Rhythms

Change is a part of life, and much of this change comes from within us. Regular fluctuations in our body chemistry produce regular rhythms or repetitions in our physiology and behavior. These rhythms are called biological rhythms. They are also called cycles, biological clocks, or just plain rhythms. In humans these cycles last from about one-tenth of a second for certain brain waves, through one second for a heartbeat and four seconds for a breath, to about twenty-eight days for the menstrual cycle (Figure 6). After the appropriate time interval, each of these events is repeated. The longest documented rhythm in nature is the flowering of a particular bamboo plant. Every hundred years (give or take a few), flowers are formed. For the lazy scientist this is the perfect thing to study, because one can always claim to be waiting for just the right moment—which can come no more than once in a lifetime. Of course, if he gets bamboozled and misses it, it would be rather embarrassing.

It is easy to see how a mechanical device such as an hourglass or wristwatch keeps time. Someone has to turn it over or wind it every so often. It is not so easy to imagine how the molecules of living cells do it. Who or what winds the clock? It seems unlikely that the biological clock that causes bamboo to flower is the same one that generates brain waves since the cycles are so different: one hundred years versus a fraction of a second. However, the important common feature all biological clocks share is their dual ability to tick away independently of any cues from the environment if need be, but also to be influenced by it at times. For example, oxygen enters our blood from the lungs when we inhale, and it is the heart's job at every beating to supply our body tissues with this oxygenated blood. The heart is beating at a steady rate independently of the environment. But as we know, events in the environment can modify the basic heart rhythm as well as our basic breathing rhythm. When we are sexually aroused or frightened, our heart beats faster and we breathe more rapidly. Our internal heartbeat clock has been reset temporarily by the environment to beat faster and pump more blood and its oxygen to the tissues that need them. When the stimulation ends, this clock soon returns to unstimulated rhythmic levels.

SEXUAL RHYTHMS   Sexual arousal in women has also been shown to be under clock control, not so much on a daily basis as over the twenty-eight day menstrual cycle. Interest in taking an active part in sexual intercourse can

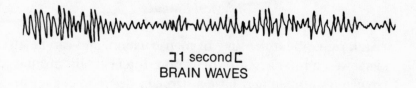

⊐ 1 second ⊏
BRAIN WAVES

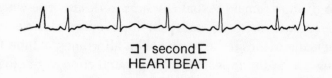

⊐ 1 second ⊏
HEARTBEAT

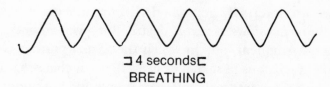

⊐ 4 seconds ⊏
BREATHING

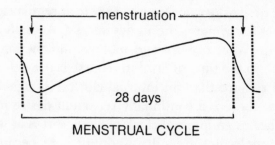

MENSTRUAL CYCLE

Figure 6: **EXAMPLES OF BIOLOGICAL CLOCKS**
Regularly reoccurring events are found in a variety of biological processes. The time between the peaks is clock controlled.

peak right about the time of menstruation, and can be at its lowest a few days after ovulation. Interestingly, around ovulation women may have a stronger desire to engage in sex, but in a much more passive way. Thus there may be two distinct female sexual rhythms in desire: one when a woman wishes to be active in intercourse and another when she wishes to be passive. Not all women exhibit this behavior, but it appears to be a general enough finding to be of interest. It is true that changes in the environment—a new man, a new location, a new whatever—may influence the internally generated rhythm, moving it to new highs or new lows of sexual desire. But given an unchanging environment, one in which the sexual partner is the same, variations in sexual desire will occur that are under the control of internal molecular events and not under the willful control of the woman.

A man, too, varies in his desire for sexual activity, but the desire does not seem to vary in as regular a fashion as it does for women—he always wants it. Actually, there is less desire after orgasm and more desire the longer it is delayed, so the time of last intercourse is the determinant of desire more than an internal clock. Nevertheless, the fact that there is a continually recurrent desire for more sex indicates an internal clock of some sort is at work. Of course, molecules are still important here because male sex-hormone chemicals (such as testosterone) influence the sexual appetite. Chemicals that directly interfere with the action of testosterone have been shown to reduce the sex drive of male habitual sex offenders. Male cancer patients who receive estrogen treatment also show a diminished sex drive.

Also under the internal clock control is the period of premenstrual tension experienced by some women. Just before menstruation, irritability, depression, or mood swings may exhibit themselves. These changes are not under the control of the woman, as they result from too-low levels of the female sex hormone progesterone as well as from other chemical changes. Evidence that hormone levels are involved in premenstrual tension comes from women taking birth-control pills, which have been found to reduce these behavioral mood swings. Men may also have cycles in mood, but they are irregular and have not been related to changes in hormonal levels.

I GOT RHYTHM, YOU GOT RHYTHM People everywhere like music, although an anthropologist will probably dig up some obscure tribe somewhere in the world that hates music. Nevertheless, music is an international language. Why is this? It has been suggested (and would it not be fascinating?) that we were all conditioned to like music in our mother's womb. This would of course have to apply to the other mammals also. Rats liked the Pied Piper's music, and cows are said to give more milk to music, so what more proof do we need? As a fetus we are surrounded by the sounds of our mother's physiology: her rhythmic heartbeat and breathing sounds. When she walks, we are also bounced rhythmically. We know a fetus can hear, as a loud sound outside will make it move. The mother's heart beats about seventy times a minute, she breathes about eighteen times a minute, and she would walk at about fifty steps (bounces) a minute. All together they would produce some interesting rhythms (including disco at 120 beats a minute). Perhaps after birth, and during the rest of our life, the rhythmic pulsations of the music we hear are sounds (in modified form) that are pleasing because we are used to hearing them. I will not go so far as to say that music reminds us of a soft, warm, peaceful place in our dear mother. I will leave this to psychiatrists to try and prove. It will be interesting to see what the response to music is from the real test-tube babies—those conceived and nurtured to full term outside the mother. If my notion is correct, their response to music should be quite different.

CIRCADIAN RHYTHMS Our internal clocks control us more than we control them. They affect us in a predictable way because their influence is rhythmic, and if we understand this, we can better understand why we do some of the things we do.

The clocks discussed thus far have produced their behavioral effects on a regular basis, as would be expected of a clock, but the events have not occurred just once a day. They either occurred more often than once a day, as with the heartbeat, or less often than every day, as with menstruation. There are rhythms, though, that occur on a daily basis, they are called circadian rhythms. Circadian means literally about a day, or about twenty-four hours. They may be the most common rhythms because they match the day-night rhythms of the earth, and these are the ones we will spend the most time with. The earth makes one complete rotation about its axis in twenty-four hours, exposing most parts of our world (the polar regions are an exception) to alternating light and dark periods.

Most of us synchronize our lives with this day-night rhythm, preferring to sleep at night and to be active during the day. But "night people" do just the opposite.

SLEEP   These so-called night people prefer to shift their activities into the night, sleeping later in the morning, while the morning people prefer early morning activity and going to bed earlier at night. While some people sleep at different times than others, we all have the same twenty-four–hour sleep-wakefulness rhythm. The time we are asleep plus the time we are awake is about twenty-four hours, and then we repeat, over and over and over again. It is reasonable to suggest that the twenty-four–hour day-night changes around us impose upon us the twenty-four–hour sleep-wakefulness rhythm. The conclusion would be that there is no internal clock producing this behavior. However, some studies of people isolated from these environmental changes have indicated that an internal clock is, indeed, present. People have volunteered to spend months in caves or isolated laboratory rooms without clocks or day-night changes. The volunteers would decide when to eat, when to turn lights on or off, and when to sleep. They were given no clues whatsoever of time passing. They were given food whenever they requested it. Yet they all showed about twenty-four–hour periods (twenty-five hours or so) of sleep-wakefulness! Their internal clock was keeping time.

Within this twenty-four–hour period there are other rhythms occurring. For example, we know that even within sleep itself there are two different states, a dream state and a nondream state. Within the nondream state are further stages of sleep ranging from the very light to the very deep. It is in the deepest stage that growth-hormone molecules are released from the brain into the bloodstream to promote body growth. As you might expect, growing children need to spend proportionally longer amounts of time in deep sleep compared to those who have reached physical maturity. Nevertheless, the total amount of time spent in sleep in cycling from the dream state to the nondream state and its stages is about ninety minutes. The relative amount of time we spend in each of the stages, however, does vary during the night. How long we sleep determines how many of these ninety-minute sleep cycles we have. As we age, we sleep less, up until our sixties, and consequently have fewer of these cycles. Beyond this age our sleep rhythms are much more variable, with some people requiring more sleep and some much less than before. In either case, older people often feel they sleep less well—the reason for this is that they spend much less total time in deep sleep.

All these sleep-cycle events are under molecular control, as is the process of sleep itself. We know, for instance, that amphetamine molecules inhibit sleep, while the molecules of anesthesia and barbiturates (sleeping pills) promote sleep. Serotonin, a naturally occurring chemical in the brain, will produce sleep when applied to certain areas of the brain; when its action is stopped, insomnia will result. In a way, the molecules that control sleep are the most important to our behavior because we do not do many interesting things in bed—that is, while we are asleep.

The Functions of Sleep Since we are awake even longer than we are asleep, it may be more meaningful to ask what is the function of being awake. Sleeping is not all that easy, for we have to get through the day first. Maybe the function of sleep is to keep us out of trouble. We can afford to sleep long, but some animals lower in the food chain—like mice and rabbits—cannot. They can best stay out of trouble by being alert and running away. We eat everything and nothing regularly eats us, tapeworms aside.

The function of sleep is probably to create a new supply of molecules to replace those that were used up while we were awake. Chemicals in the body are being continually used up and need to be replenished. Those who need less sleep may just require less time to resynthesize the molecules they have used up. All our activities require chemicals, whether we are thinking, moving about, or just maintaining body functions such as our heartbeat and breathing rate. The ultimate source of these chemicals is of course food, which is broken down and separated by the digestive system into water, vitamins, minerals, proteins, carbohydrates, fats, and nucleic acids (chemicals of the genes). These are used by the body either as they are or broken down into even smaller molecules (proteins into amino acids, for example), to be rebuilt into new molecules peculiar to the needs of humans. The proteins we get from foods do not have the same chemical structure as the proteins we need for our own body. Therefore, our digestive enzymes break down food protein into its component parts—amino acids—and then our body uses these amino acids to make different proteins having the proper chemical structure for our own body. During wakefulness we apparently cannot keep up with the demand our body has upon molecules. The body has its own energy crisis. Sleep gives us the opportunity to meet this crisis.

It has been shown that many chemicals are made in greater abundance during sleep than during wakefulness. Furthermore, our brain uses no less oxygen during sleep than during wakefulness, indicating the brain is not chemically at rest when the remainder of our body is. It may also be that we sleep more during colds and the flu in order to give our body more time to repair tissue damage resulting from these infections.

Given these functions of sleep, it is not surprising that sleep deprivation seriously affects our behavior. Prolonged sleep deprivation in animals has been shown to cause death—the ultimate disruption of behavior. More commonly, the lack of sleep leads to irritability, the inability to concentrate, and to less coordinated body movements. If the right molecules are not in the right place at the right time, these behavioral problems arise.

DREAMS We all dream, and this must have some significance, as dreams are not just random thought patterns. They have a story line and progress from one event to another. We dream as we think, and do not dream in letters of the alphabet or in nonsense words. The dream state can be ascertained in the laboratory by certain brain-wave patterns (recorded from the scalp) and rapid back-and-forth eye movements, visible when the eyelids are lifted. In the laboratory, if awakened right after a dream, most people can recall that dream. However, upon awakening naturally at the end of a night's sleep, at home or elsewhere, a person may be able to remember that a dream occurred, but would not know exactly when it occurred or how many dreams there were. There often are several dreams a night, but usually only the last one is remembered, if that. As much as ninety percent of our dreams may not be remembered. The purpose of dreams is not then to make us aware of all our unconscious brain activity, or most dreams would be remembered. It has not been demonstrated that the ten percent of dreams that get through are more important to us than the ninety percent that do not.

Since biblical times, and possibly earlier, dreams have been thought to have hidden meanings. In the Book of Genesis, for example, the Pharaoh says to Joseph, "I have heard it said of you that when you hear a dream you can interpret it." Much later, Sigmund Freud and his contemporaries said that dreams also perform an important, useful function for the dreamer. Dreams, it was said, bring to our awareness suppressed wishes in disguised form that the dreams fulfill or attempt to fulfill. Freud felt the dream was couched (get it?) in mystery. The dream needs to be interpreted to determine what the wish really is, and the interpretation helps to understand a wide range of behaviors. Unfortunately, proper interpretations now start at fifty dollars or more per hour. There are many bodily processes (such as blood-cell production and the breakdown of proteins into amino acids) that go on without our awareness. There is no reason either why the brain could not conduct some of its business in secret and not reveal to us what dreams are all about.

The Meaning of Dreams • How can we know for sure the meaning of dreams? There are those who believe that the objects in dreams are only representations of something else. If a group of people believe that caves and boxes in dreams represent vaginas, and cigars and poles represent penises, this still does not constitute proof—it is an opinion. For a while, everyone believed the sun rotated about the earth. This was not proof, it was an opinion also. Surely there must be times in a dream, as Freud would admit, when "a cigar was just a cigar." A belief does not constitute a scientific proof. To prove something requires that alternative explanations can be ruled out, and this has not been done in dream analysis. There is no limit to the number of ways dreams can be interpreted.

Consider the following analogy. A metal box (a wish) is buried underground (in our unconsciousness). We do not know how the box (or the wish) got there, or even if it is there to begin with. We walk along with a metal detector (a part of our brain) and it beep-beeps (dreams). The beep-beep (dreams) represent the box (wish) in a disguised form. Other metallic objects (thoughts that are not wishes) could also produce the beep-beeps (dreams), so we do not know exactly what the beep-beeps represent. The only way to find out is to dig up what is producing the beep-beep sound. Unfortunately we cannot put our fingers on what is producing the dream. Analogies do not prove a point, they only illustrate it, and the point is that we cannot yet determine what the content of a dream represents. Anyone can interpret a dream; no one can prove it is the correct interpretation.

Things often happen in dreams that do not happen when we are awake. We may dream of sexual activity, physical violence, and other things that we would never consider doing when awake. These might be just tangled-up thoughts and memories generated by the data processing in our brains. Or we may dream about things that trouble us, in an attempt to solve these problems in some way. But since our unconscious is unknown to us, by definition, how can we say that dreams or anything else reveal it to us? Another possibility is that dreams tie together thoughts about our daily lives with past events in our memory (how molecules represent memories will be covered in the next chapter). That is, day-to-day events are accommodated within our memories by the act of dreaming. We also do this, of course, to a much greater extent while we are awake, so dreaming merely extends this process. Severely retarded people appear to dream less. Those who have lost their speech temporarily (by a blow to the head or a stroke) dream more at night while working during the day to regain their speech than those who have lost their speech permanently.

As we all know, what goes on in our dreams in one way or another reflects what is going on in our lives. Dreams often have people and places in them that we know. So what we do influences a dream to some extent. It is possible, however, to influence a dream directly, as laboratory studies with humans have shown. When shown films with a high emotional content (people being hurt, for instance), some people will report that their dreams included some action contained within the film. Even more impressive are experiments where red goggles are worn before going to sleep. Here, some people report having red-tinted dreams. These experiments indicate in a dramatic way that the world around us finds its way into our dreams and our molecules.

For whatever reason dreaming occurs, its presence does serve to stimulate our nervous system and keep it active. It has been found that the human fetus (near full term) spends more than fifty percent of its total sleep time dreaming. A newborn spends about fifty percent of its sleep time dreaming, decreasing to about twenty-five percent by age five, where it stays fairly constant until old age, declining then to eighteen percent or less. One cannot help but conclude that dreaming has some role in the development and maintenance of our nervous system.

It is known that when people are deprived of dreaming by being awakened as soon as a dream starts, they have more dreams when they go back to sleep. It is as though the brain is making up for any dreaming loss. On the other hand, depriving someone of dreaming does not seem to have any effect upon their behavior when awake. If awakened during dreaming, one becomes irritable, as laboratory studies show. But people are usually irritable when awakened, whether they were dreaming or not. More significantly, when people are deprived of dream sleep with certain drugs for several days or even for as long as six months, no gross changes in behavior result. They behave just as "sanely" as those allowed to dream. Over the short run, then, dreams are not necessary to our well-being as adults. Psychological theories that suggest dreams are crucial to our emotional life must be seriously questioned.

RHYTHMS IN PERFORMANCE   It is said we will be more the same person tomorrow at this time than we will be later today. This is another effect of our internal circadian rhythms. Twenty-four hours from now our body will be performing at the same levels as it is now, but in a few hours from now new performance levels will reach their peaks and others will diminish. If we are typing, sorting papers, or driving a car, for example, there will be certain times of the day when we can do them better. Just about any job we do, we can do better at certain times of the day. Similarly, there will be a time of the day when we perform a task at our worst, doing it more slowly or less accurately. Of course, external events can affect our performance levels also. A cup of coffee, a meal, or a brief change of scenery can perk us up; boredom can slow us down. But the basic rhythm is generated within us.

Ideally, a company would match its work schedules to the performance rhythms of the employees. Only a few organizations around the world have done this, because of the obvious difficulty of rearranging work schedules on an individual basis, while still maintaining coordination of effort among employees. Where accomplished, the results have been promising. On-the-job accidents have been reduced and productivity has increased because people are working at their best possible body times. This has been achieved by measuring the actual speed and accuracy in doing a job over a several-day period. Each worker's job schedule was matched as closely as possible to the peak performance times. It was not accomplished astrologically by computing forward from birth times and somehow estimating the best performance times from this. This is popularly known as the biorhythms approach, which deals with physical, intellectual, and emotional rhythms.

Unfortunately, the computation of biorhythms takes no account of either the genetic makeup of an individual (which generates the rhythms) or environmental influences (which can modify the rhythms) such as a changed sleeping schedule. Since both these factors are the only determinants of rhythmic behavior, their absence in a biorhythm computation leaves nothing of value. No one has yet been able to demonstrate a causal relationship between time of birth and subsequent circadian rhythms of any sort. By chance a biorhythm prediction may agree from time to time with your assessment of how you feel. There is also a kind of circular thinking that develops. For whatever reason, if you want to believe in biorhythms, then you will find something in your feelings each day that will agree with the biorhythm prediction. If you do not want to believe in biorhythms, then you will deny that your feelings on any day agree with the biorhythm prediction. In short, the molecules of our brain will often not let in information from the environment that will change the existing molecular structure. This is called resistance to change.

It is as though the molecular gods are playing in our body. When they are abundant and energetic, they work harder and we perform better; and when they are scarce and weakened, they do not work as hard and our performance is at its worst. Scientifically speaking, those molecular interactions that eventually translate into our ability to perform a task are being modified or controlled by an internal molecular clock. It has been shown, for instance, that our performance rhythms are related quite directly to our body-temperature rhythms. Body temperature is not at all constant at 98.6°F, but varies rhythmically over twenty-four hours by as much as two degrees.* It so happens that when temperature peaks, our performance often does too. Figure 7 illustrates this relationship. The efficiency with which we do our work varies rhythmically over a twenty-four–hour period, with different people reaching their most efficient performance at different times. It is not known for sure, but it is quite possible that the body-temperature changes produce the performance changes. We saw in chapter 1 that molecules move about more as the temperature increases. Increased molecular motion could put more molecules at the right place faster, thereby increasing the efficiency of our muscles and facilitating the movement of molecules across nerve-cell membranes in our brain to help us think faster.

DRUGS, INFECTIONS, AND DEATH   Our responsiveness to drugs is also under internal-clock control. Drugs are molecules (some would say a drug can be defined as

---

*You can check this out yourself. With an oral thermometer, take your temperature for a couple of days every four hours or so—at night too, if you wake up. Do it before sex, jogging, or other exercises, as these raise the body temperature temporarily. You should find regular fluctuations in your temperature. See if your peak body temperature corresponds to your high point of the day. If it does not, forget I mentioned it.

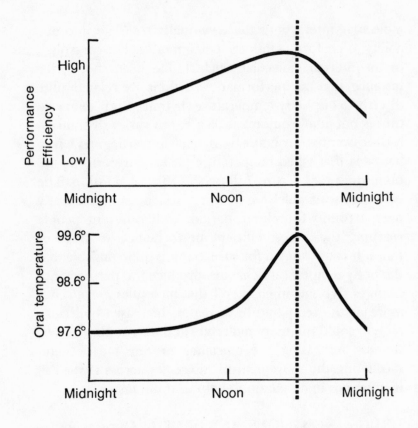

Figure 7: **TEMPERATURE
AND PERFORMANCE RHYTHMS**
*Body temperature (lower curve) peaks at the same time of day
that performance (upper curve) peaks. The shape of the curves
would vary with the individual. In this case, both body
temperature and the efficiency of performing a task peak at
about six* P.M.

any chemical that has a five hundred percent price markup) and their interaction with other molecules in the body under clock control produces a variety of behavioral effects. The responses of animals to several drugs, including amphetamines, alcohol, and anesthetics, vary according to the time of day they are administered. When rats were given a large dose of amphetamine at the end of what would be their notion of daytime, only a small number of them died. But given the same dose during the middle of their day, nearly eighty percent were killed. Similar experiments with alcohol and mice demonstrated changing susceptibility over the day to lethal doses of this drug. Human studies have shown that alcohol is metabolized at different rates at different times of the day. We can hold our liquor better in the afternoon and evening than in the early morning hours. The enzyme molecules in the body chew up alcohol much more readily from about noon to midnight, resulting in less alcohol in the blood and reduced intoxicating effects. The extent of our drunken behavior is determined by internal molecular events acting on the alcohol we drink. Other ways in which our internal physiology plays a role in alcoholism will be discussed in chapter 6. In addition, morning surgical operations are not optimally matched to our anesthesia sensitivity, as a larger and more dangerous dose is needed in the morning compared to the afternoon. Early morning surgery does free the physician, though, for afternoon golf, and real estate deals.

Antihistamine treatment of allergies has been shown to be more effective in the duration of its effect in the morning than in the evening. Aspirin, too, is more effective, for any given dose, when given in the morning. On the other hand, people allergic to penicillin show the greatest sensitivity to it late in the evening. While not all drugs have been studied, it is a safe bet that the effect of most drugs is influenced by our molecular rhythms.

We are susceptible not only to rhythmic drug effects but also to rhythmic infection patterns. The larval form of the microorganism responsible for elephantiasis (a grotesque enlargement of the leg or scrotum) leaves the bloodstream during the day and moves into the lungs, then back again the next day, repeating this cycle during the course of the infection. Animal studies have shown that injections of disease-causing bacteria will produce death at certain times of the day, but not at others. Experiments like this cannot be done on humans, but the parallels between animal and human rhythms are strong enough to suggest that humans would respond like animals.

Infectious microorganisms (bacteria, fungi, protozoa, roundworms, and viruses) probably have a better chance of infecting us at certain times of our circadian rhythms than at other times when our physiological defenses are not at their peak. It has been observed that bacterial infections (such as tonsillitis, appendicitis, and pneumonia) start more frequently in the morning, as contrasted to viral infections (such as influenza) which start more frequently in the evening. Death from a variety of causes occurs most frequently from four to six A.M., and births peak at about the same time, two to four A.M. Early in the morning our heartbeat-rate rhythm is at a minimum and may be most amenable to disruption and failure. We know that some hormone levels in the body vary in a circadian manner; early in the morning those involved in initiating birth may be at maximal levels.

SENSORY RESPONSIVENESS   Does a member of the opposite sex always look so good, smell so good, and sound so good throughout the day? Probably not, because our biological rhythms influence our sensory impressions also. From about five to seven P.M. our senses may be at their peak. What we like may seem at its best then, while what we dislike will appear at its worst. Traffic noises and the yelling of children may seem unusually irritating at this time, while the cat or dog we come home to looks pretty good and food smells and tastes particularly fine.

The intensity of the pain and pleasure we experience may also be under clock control. We know our teeth are the most sensitive to pain during the time of dentists' office hours. The only comforting news here is that the extreme peak of pain sensitivity may be around six P.M., when the office is closed. It is not surprising that if our senses peak at about this time, our sensitivity to pain would also peak then. There are identifiable pleasure centers in animal brains which can be electrically stimulated to give them pleasure. Animals easily learn to press levers or buttons to self-administer stimulation if their brains have been wired up in the laboratory to receive it. While the animals stimulate themselves throughout twenty-four hours, most stimulation occurs in the evening. This suggests a rhythm in pleasure sensitivity which humans might also possess.

It may be that everything entering our senses is

subject to the rhythmic fluctuations of our senses and nervous system. We may learn faster and remember better at some times of the day than at others. A particular situation may be more fearsome at one time than another. We may respond better with all our senses to another person at certain times of the day, and we may be less troubled by what is happening at certain times of the day. Our molecules that make up the biological clock are dictating to us how we feel and act, although we may have expected to behave pretty much the same throughout the day.

RHYTHMS IN MOOD We also experience mood swings during the day that reflect not only how our senses are responding, but also what our body temperature is. We may be more cheerful and friendly, for example, as the day progresses, up until the time our body temperature reaches its maximum. From then on it is downhill, and we become less cheerful, possibly even grouchy. Events of the day will affect our moods also—they cannot help but have an effect—but they will be superimposed over our internal body rhythms. We know that stressful events will have the biggest effect on our rhythms. When stressed, we often cannot sleep or eat because our sleep and hunger rhythms have been knocked out of kilter.

RESETTING OUR CLOCKS In the discussion above, the time at which certain behaviors peak has been based on the assumption that we are following the most common schedule of sleep and wakefulness, where we sleep at night and are active during the day. Our twenty-four–hour rhythms are set according to this schedule. If we change our schedule to sleep during the day and to be active at night, our circadian rhythms will—over a period of a few days—be reset by our new schedule. Our sensory responses will then peak at new times, shifted by as many hours as our schedule has been shifted. For example, if we go to sleep about eleven P.M., our senses peak as we have seen at about six P.M. If we shift our sleep twelve hours to go to bed at eleven A.M., our sensory peak will shift twelve hours also to peak at six A.M. The number of days it takes to accomplish this shift in our biological rhythm goes by the modern name of jet lag, because jets move us rapidly across time zones. No one ever heard of wagon-train lag.

In view of the rhythms in our behavior, it is not surprising that moving quickly into quite different time zones has an unfavorable effect upon our behavior. On the average it takes about one-half to one day per one-hour time change to purge oneself of jet lag. During this adjustment time we just cannot be operating at the peak of all our rhythms. Business deals may be mishandled, athletic events performed less well, and sightseeing made less pleasurable. We may stay up some nights so that we do not have a circadian rhythm (we could sleep four hours and be awake twelve hours—a sixteen hour rhythm), but this will not last long before our internally generated twenty-four–hour rhythm predominates. We will eventually sleep long enough to get back into a twenty-four–hour sleep-wakefulness rhythm. The twenty-four–hour rhythm will persist because there is a genetic basis for it. Our genes are programmed to produce this twenty-four–hour rhythm, as well as many other circadian ones. Experiments with plants and animals that possess twenty-four–hour rhythms have shown that the production of mutations in the genes is the only way to change the length of these rhythms permanently. Chemicals and X rays can produce mutations in the genes involved in the timekeeping process. With these treatments, some twenty-four–hour rhythms in plants and animals have been changed to as short as fifteen hours and as long as forty hours. These are permanent changes that will last as long as the organism does.

While gene-mutation experiments such as these cannot, obviously, be done on humans for ethical reasons, it is certainly possible that a few of us carry within ourselves gene mutations of our sleep-wakefulness rhythms so that we do not function on a twenty-four–hour rhythm. We are not talking of someone who sleeps five hours a day and is active nineteen hours, for this is still a twenty-four–hour cycle. A noncircadian rhythm would mean someone is sleeping, say, five hours a day, but is active only fifteen hours a day (twenty-hour rhythm) or active twenty-three hours a day (twenty-eight–hour rhythm). These rhythms would be genetically normal for them, but they would be out of synchronization with everyone else's approximately twenty-four–hour rhythm. This is really marching to the beat of a different drummer, and one would suspect that this would produce behavior problems for noncircadian persons. The expectations of people around them as to when is the proper time to sleep, to eat, and to be active would not be matched by noncircadian persons. They could well feel different and out of place, with their behavior reflecting this. Less severe changes in the sleep-wakefulness rhythm are symptomatic of certain illnesses. For example the severely depressed often suffer from insomnia. Depressed people can sometimes be temporarily brought out of depression by having them go to sleep (and arising) six hours earlier than usual. Resetting their sleep-wakefulness clock puts it back in synchronization with the clocks controlling mood swings and body temperature to reestablish a normal balance.

AIRPLANE ACCIDENTS AND RHYTHMS   For most of us jet lag is an inconvenience, but for others like airplane pilots it can be a life-or-death matter. If we are on their airplane, it is for us too. It is estimated that over half of airplane accidents are due to pilot error and not mechanical failure of the airplane. For commercial pilots who regularly fly through various time zones, one can easily imagine that disrupted circadian rhythms of wakefulness, mood, performance, and sensory awareness will not be at optimal levels. It is not easy to prove these problems are the cause of accidents, however. How can we be sure that a misjudged distance, a misread dial, or a mistouched control was caused by rhythm problems? Clearly the pilot was not performing well if pilot error caused an accident, but the pilot could just have been careless. Commercial pilots particularly follow rather strict procedures in flying, and the routine of one flight after another could lead to boredom and carelessness. Regardless of the cause of pilot error, we can assume pilots do not crash on purpose, so molecular events in their bodies are not under their control. A good guess is that it *is* the molecular events of circadian rhythms that are to blame, since boredom and carelessness are more likely to occur when sensory awareness and performance are not at their peaks.

CLOCK DRUGS   The use of drugs called chronobiotics to eliminate jet lag is a timely development. Experiments on the body-temperature rhythm of rats have demonstrated this is possible. During the early part of their circadian rhythm, the depressant drug phenobarbitol can set back the temperature rhythm several hours so it will peak earlier. Similarly, during the later part of the rhythm, the stimulant drug theophylline can advance the temperature rhythm up to several hours. While all possible rhythms have not been changed, this is a beginning. One can imagine taking an appropriate chronobiotic (a "time syrup") while traveling across time zones to eliminate jet lag. Such a drug would move our mood, sensory, performance, and sleep-wakefulness rhythms forward if moving eastward (the east is always ahead of the west), or backward if moving westward. It would make our internal clocks correspond to the external clock of where we are going. Once we have a molecular understanding of the clock, we may be able to select just certain rhythms to change for a short time. We may wish to be at a sensory peak during dinner, a mood peak for that special person, and an intellectual peak for income-tax audits.

THE TICKING OF OUR CLOCKS   While it has been relatively easy to document rhythmic behavioral fluctuations, it has not been easy to identify the molecules responsible. One theory of how our circadian clock ticks involves our genetic material DNA (*d*eoxyribo*n*ucleic *a*cid). The genes of all plants and animals are composed of DNA. Within the structure of these very large molecules (the largest molecules in our body) is encoded all the necessary information to make and operate an organism. The DNA determines not only our body structure and sex, but also exerts control over our bodily processes. Segments of the DNA molecules in our cells are separated into genes, and there are at least fifty thousand genes per human cell, perhaps as many as five hundred thousand. Essentially, every cell contains a copy of all our genes, except that some genes are always turned off. For instance, a brain cell does not "need or want" to be a liver cell, so the genes that make a cell a liver cell are turned off. Likewise, a liver cell turns off those genes that could turn it into a brain cell.

Each behavior under clock control may have a gene (piece of DNA) influencing it. The information from the genes (which are located in the nucleus of each cell) is transferred one gene at a time to another molecule called messenger RNA (*r*ibo*n*ucleic *a*cid). The messenger RNA molecule leaves the nucleus of the cell and moves into the cytoplasm (see Figure 8), where it attaches to a very small structure in the cell called a ribosome. Here the messenger RNA molecule directs the assembly of a protein. This protein is the unique product of a particular gene. That is, each gene is responsible for the production of one kind of protein. Since DNA is our genetic substance, its structure must be protected at all times, and it is protected best in the nucleus or center of a cell. This is why the DNA does not itself leave the nucleus to move to a ribosome in the cytoplasm to make protein, and then move back to the nucleus. During the trip, DNA could be damaged, and we would suffer for it. By making a copy of itself in the form of messenger RNA, the DNA protects itself and puts the risk on the messenger. If the messenger gets destroyed somehow, the DNA can send another one to the ribosome.

The ribosome acts as the workbench upon which the complex assembly of proteins occurs; when the protein is assembled, it leaves the ribosome. Proteins are composed of amino acids, of which there are twenty-two varieties. These twenty-two different amino acids may be strung together on the ribosome in any combination from just a few up to hundreds of thousands. But which combination is assembled is specified by the messenger RNA, which copies the DNA's instructions. By no means are all possible combinations used by a cell. If there are fifty thousand genes in each of our cell's DNA, then each cell can make only fifty thousand different proteins. But as we saw, not all of them are needed at once.

A gene may make only one copy of a specific protein or millions of copies, depending upon what the situation calls for. In the case of a clock gene, a few copies of one protein could be made every twenty-four hours per cell. Only those cells in a particular part of the body would be involved for any particular rhythm. If we are talking about a circadian rhythm in taste sensitivity, for example, only those cells in the taste buds need be involved. One could imagine that proteins are assembled in taste-bud cells under the direction of a clock gene for taste. These proteins would move just outside of the taste-bud cells, where they would fit alongside the recesses food molecules fit into (see chapter 1, Figure 4). This extra bit of protein could facilitate the development of nerve impulses from the taste buds to the brain (by allowing atoms and molecules to move more quickly across membranes) to heighten the taste of food for the few hours the protein remains. After a few hours, the protein molecule could self-destruct (shake itself apart with the motion given it by body heat) and taste-bud sensitivity would return to normal. Twenty-four hours later, the process would repeat itself, and so on.

Rhythms in other sensory processes would work similarly. By this theory, the other circadian rhythms we have discussed would also depend upon particular proteins being assembled at the right time every twenty-four hours, followed by their destruction a few hours later, depending upon how long a behavior was at its peak. Each rhythm would probably have its own unique protein which would cause the behavioral fluctuation. Rhythms occurring less frequently would have genes directing protein assembly less frequently. These are only guesses about how our clocks function, but we know molecules must be involved.

AGING: PROGRAMMED SELF-DESTRUCTION Every species has its own unique life span: A dog does not exceed 35 years, a horse 50, or a human 140, for example, because their self-destruction is built into their molecular structure! The fact that each kind of animal must die before a certain time has elapsed indicates the presence of some kind of "death clock." Such a clock runs down, and when it stops, we stop—permanently. Death during old age comes from a variety of diseases and organ failures, to

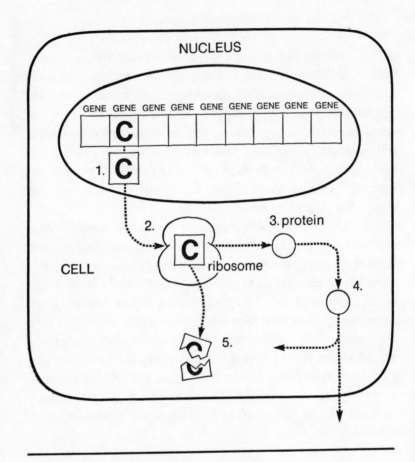

Figure 8: HOW A BIOLOGICAL
CLOCK MAY WORK
*A clock gene in the DNA of a cell is copied by a messenger
RNA molecule (1). This molecule moves out of the cell nucleus
to the ribosome (2) where it directs the assembly of a protein
molecule (3). The protein can stay inside the cell ultimately to
affect behavior or it can move outside to affect another cell (4).
When the messenger RNA molecule is finished making its
protein, it is destroyed (5).*

be sure, but something always gets us before we reach 140 years. Something is limiting our life span, and it is not environmental. People are living longer now because of health-care improvements, but the maximum age we reach has probably not changed since our species evolved, about forty thousand years ago. Our environment has changed much since then. Our life span is therefore built into our molecular structure.

We may mechanically just wear out until our vital organs fail. Were they to have a different molecular structure, they would wear out after a different time period—maybe sooner, maybe later—and our life span would vary accordingly. By this theory of aging, our ultimate time of death is built into our molecular structures. Other theories of aging suggest the process is more direct, resulting from actual aging genes. These genes would be a form of clock gene which would be turned on after a certain age was reached. The genes would synthesize proteins (see Figure 8) that would actually function to shut down bodily processes. Normally, any aging genes we have could be activated by our thirties (when many of our processes start to show decline) with the harmful effects accumulating until we are done in. A medical disorder called Cockayne syndrome suggests that aging genes may actually exist. This is a genetic abnormality described first by a London physician, Dr. Cockayne. It is not one of the world's pressing problems, as only some thirty-odd cases have been reported. It is a disease of premature senility that is seen in children as young as six or seven! They appear normal as infants, but by six or seven they show clear signs of old age: deafness, vision problems, muscle weakness, wrinkled skin, bad teeth, tremor of the hands, and general uncoordinated movements. It is as though the aging genes were turned on way too soon.

Why should we age and die anyhow? If we have genes to prevent us from living essentially forever, then there must be some benefit to dying for those who remain living. One can only guess as to purpose in nature. One guess about dying would be that if all animals, including us, lived essentially forever and continued reproducing they would run out of food. Some would therefore die, and living forever would be impossible anyhow. By having a sort of programmed death in the molecules of our genes (so that we will die eventually even if no one eats or kills us), there is a better guarantee for a continual food supply for those who survive.

Our genes determine which of our behaviors are under clock control. Those that are, fluctuate in intensity over time. Most of our biological rhythms are circadian (occurring every twenty-four hours) to match the natural light-dark cycle of our environment. A few rhythms may occur more frequently or less frequently. The twenty-four–hour period is determined genetically, since only gene mutations can change this. Within this twenty-four–hour period we can shift our various rhythms to peak at different times by changing our sleep-wakefulness cycle. But we can do nothing to stop the rhythmic occurrences of those behaviors, as they are internally generated. We are changing involuntarily. Our behavior changes from hour to hour because of the location and structure of our molecules.

3

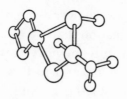

Thinking

A powerful force is at work inside our brain. The force is with us and it is molecular. We saw in Chapter 1 that the people, places, things, and events of our environment are translated into molecular events by our senses. After it passes through our senses, the molecular representation of the environment will either be ignored or stored in our memory. Our brain does not utilize everything around us that our senses are exposed to. For example, we can walk into a room and look around at its contents, but if asked what we saw, we may remember only a few objects in the room. It is possible, however, that everything we saw or heard, smelled, touched, or tasted in that room was stored in our brain, even though we could not remember it all.

In theory, the human brain could store one hundred billion pieces of information, because there are that many nerve cells in the brain. The assumption is that each nerve cell in our brain could store one piece of information by slightly modifying its chemical structure. To get this much information into our brain, our senses would have to take in about seventy-five pieces of information every second we are awake over our entire lifetime. This is probably more information than we actually take in, so our brain is never at its full memory capacity. Everyone is capable of learning more, and in this sense no one ever uses his or her brain to the maximum extent possible. "You are never too old to learn" makes more biological sense than "You can't teach an old dog new tricks." For comparison, there is no computer the size of the human brain that can store this much information. Computers are also expensive to produce. As pointed out the human brain and the body that carries it around, on the other hand, are mass produced by unskilled labor, for free.

In spite of our potential to store everything in our brain that we experience, it is not clear why we would want to do so, since most of us do not make good use of the information we have! The alternative to storing everything we experience is for new information to replace old information, up to a point. Modern electronic calculators can illustrate the differences between these two types of memory storage. When adding numbers, the sum is displayed on the calculator. For simple calculators, adding together another set of numbers produces a new sum that replaces the previous one, which is then gone (forgotten) forever. The more advanced calculators, however, will store previous sums in other memories as new sums are produced. Eventually, all these memories will be used up too, as we perform more additions. Theoretically, as we have seen, the brain may never use up all its memories, but what happens in practice we do not know. To make room for new memories, some old ones may have to disappear. A professor who taught a botany course was once criticized by his students for not remembering their names. He replied that for every name of theirs he remembered, he forgot the name of a plant. This is going too far, as no one has ever learned as much as he or she possibly can. It is more likely that a selection process (our interest, if you will) is somehow operating to limit the amount of information flowing into memory. Most of our sensory input is simply not important enough to be stored for future use; the remaining sensory input, however, goes into short-term memory, and then possibly into long-term memory, as Figure 9 shows.

Short-term memory, as the name implies, does not last very long. Someone gives us a telephone number to call; after dialing it, we forget it. With frequent use, this same number would find its way into long-term memory. Practice (repetition) converts short-term memory into long-term memory. The actual use of the telephone number to produce the behavior of dialing we would call thinking. For purposes of definition, thinking is data processing. As Figure 9 indicates, environmental information in short-term memory is either used right away in thinking or placed in long-term memory or forgotten. Information stored in long-term memory may last as long as we do, may be used in thinking, or may be eventually forgotten. The thinking process may lead to some action on our part, or be used to develop thought that can be stored in either short-term or long-term memory. How often do we think of something and then forget it? It has gone into short-term memory and then was forgotten. How often do we almost remember something, but cannot quite get it? The memory has not been retrieved from storage.

Figure 9 is a model or representation of how thinking relates to information about our environment as processed by our senses. Without this input from our environment, our thinking would not amount to much at all, as we would have no experiences to trouble or please us, no facts to assemble into thoughts, and nothing to reflect on and plan with. As you might expect, the retrieval of information is much more complex than Figure 9 indicates. We know that we can remember something better if the memory is associated with something else we know. An example some use is to ask you to remember the number 200117761984. It may take a little time. If asked to remember a number that represents the name of a science-fiction motion picture, the date of the founding of the United States and the title of a novel by George Orwell, it would be much easier to remember because the numbers are now associated with something else.

SHORT-TERM MEMORY   The components of Figure 9 have a molecular basis to them. The nerve impulses produced by the senses may serve by themselves as the basis for short-term memory. What we sense around us is coded into specific patterns of nerve impulses which represent the memory. As we saw in chapter 1, the nerve impulses are created by atomic and molecular movements moving across nerve-cell membranes. A conversation, the

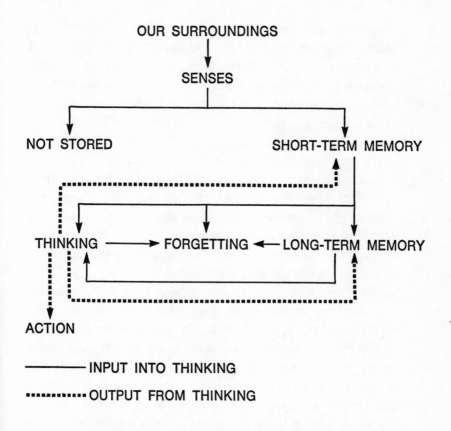

Figure 9: **BRAIN WORK**
This diagram shows the interrelationship of thinking and memory, and how both are influenced by what our senses take in from our surroundings.

feel of a thigh, a glance at a person—all will be represented by a specific pattern of nerve impulses. The pattern of impulses for these events moves from our senses through thousands or millions of nerve cells until the senses have conveyed their message to specific regions of the brain. This is a very quick trip, for within a tenth of a second our brain receives the message representing a sound, smell, taste, touch, or image. As long as these impulses last in our brain, short-term memory will last. The longer these impulses last, the greater the chance that long-term memory will develop. We can make this happen by thinking about what we have experienced or by repeating the actual experience. We may see something only once for a brief moment; it goes into short-term memory. If we think about what we just saw because we want to remember it, then we can move it to long-term memory. The other way to remember it (to get it into long-term memory) is to look at it for a relatively long time. Let me give you an example. You want to see a famous art museum but do not have much time, so you dash through all the galleries, looking at hundreds of pictures. Most of these pictures will not get past short-term memory—they will be forgotten. Those you particularly like, you will think about, and this repetition in the brain will lead to long-term memory for these pictures. Repetition leads to remembering. In principle, developing a habit (good or bad) is no different. We repeat a behavior often enough so that it goes into long-term memory, where it becomes difficult to get rid of.

Our short-term memory is rather delicate and is easily disrupted by a blow to the head, for example. This is probably because the nerve impulses carrying the short-term memory have not yet been consolidated into more permanent molecular structures. Nerve impulses are essentially electrical events produced, as we have seen, by the flow across nerve-cell membranes of molecules and atoms which possess either positive or negative electrical charges. Continually moving from nerve cell to nerve cell, these electrical events are easily disturbed. With a break in the proper pattern of events, the memory represented by them is lost. Electrical shocks applied to the brain will eliminate short-term memory but not long-term memory. That is, things recently learned will be forgotten, but not things learned long ago. Presumably, the applied electricity disrupts the brain's internal electrical events, essentially producing short circuits in short-term memory patterns. Long-term memory is not affected because it exists in a different form.

LONG-TERM MEMORY While short-term memory may last from seconds to hours, long-term memory lasts from days to years—often a lifetime. Long-term memories may be represented by a persistent pattern of nerve impulses moving through a large number of nerve-cell pathways without disappearing as they do in short-term memory. Something in the brain allows these patterns to continue uninterrupted, perhaps by moving them to new pathways in the brain. When a thought crosses our mind, it may do just that. Another guess as to how long-term memories are represented is that the pattern of nerve impulses, produced in short-term memory, causes the synthesis of memory molecules or a change in the chemical structure of preexisting molecules that make up part of the nerve cells. For simplicity of discussion, let us just consider the molecular changes. These molecular changes would take place in a large number of brain nerve cells, probably where one cell connects with another. These connections would determine the particular nerve-cell pathways used. There might be the same changes in each nerve cell, or each nerve cell might have a different molecular change. In this latter case, no one nerve cell would have a complete memory, for a complete memory could only be obtained by the participation of all the cells having a part of the memory. It is as though the complete memory was for a word, but each nerve-cell connection only had one letter of it.

The production of memory molecules would imply that every memory was represented by a particular molecule or group of molecules. A molecule representing the memory for a tree, for instance, would have a different shape than the memory molecule for a sports car. If we remember a particularly comfortable chair our parents had when we were a child, many memory molecules would be necessary to represent not only the concept of a chair, but also its color, texture, location in a room, and its comfort. Similar things may be represented by similar molecules since similar things would produce similar nerve impulses in our senses. The similar nerve impulses would produce similar molecular changes to produce the long-term memory. For example, when we look at someone's face, our eye codes a picture of that face into the nerve-impulse language. These nerve impulses, it is suggested, can produce molecular changes in nerve cells that represent long-term memory. When we look at another person's face, it will have similar enough properties to any other face to produce similar nerve impulses. Similar nerve impulses will then generate similar memory molecules. Therefore, each type of object—faces, trees, cars, fences, etc.—will produce a certain type of general nerve impulse to represent it.

There could be just one memory molecule for each thing we remember. More likely, there would be many copies, and molecules representing a particular memory would be scattered throughout parts of the brain, connected by nerve-impulse pathways. We know from surgical operations that a great deal of the brain has to be removed before there is a serious loss of memory. Pushing back the foreskin of our ignorance a bit, we might say that any form of memory storage would produce the same effect in the brain. The effect would be that the flow of charged atoms and molecules (which produce the nerve impulses) across nerve-cell membranes would be facilitated. The faster flow of atoms and molecules would mean that nerve impulses would move faster in the brain, and faster impulses signify learning. If we have learned something, we respond more quickly. After we have learned arithmetic, adding the numbers six plus four takes virtually no time at all.

MEMORY RECALL AND FORGETTING One can imagine, in theory, how molecules and electrical events in nerve cells encode our memories, but it has been far more difficult to propose a specific way in which these memories can be recalled. Generally, the best one can do is to suggest that remembering is the reverse process of learning. Nerve impulses generated by the senses may ultimately produce memory molecules. For us to recall this information coded into molecules, memory molecules may reverse the process by somehow generating another kind of nerve impulse, which carries with it the information stored in the molecule. When we cannot remember something right away, when it is on the tip of our tongue (more likely on the tip of our brain nerve cells), the memory molecules are somehow not accessible to recall.

The actual number of our nerve cells does not seem to decrease very much at all over our lifetime, so forgetting cannot merely be due to the loss of nerve cells. More likely, forgetting involves the destruction of memory molecules. The older the memory molecule, the longer it would be subject to other molecules banging into it (remember that our body heat causes molecules to bounce about), with the greater likelihood it would be destroyed. This would account for older memories fading, because the molecules are fading. Older people often do not remember things that just happened to them or things they just did. This is not because these recent memory molecules have decayed, but because these recent events never reached long-term memory to begin with. In old age, the transformation of nerve impulses into long-term molecular changes is not proceeding properly. It is not that the elderly forgot something, but that they never remembered something in the first place.

There is always the possibility (with the elderly or anybody else) that some memories have not decayed but simply have become irretrievable from storage. The memories are there, but we cannot get to them. There is some evidence that older mice can remember as well as younger mice if given diets rich in the chemicals lecithin or choline. These chemicals may lead to the increased production of acetylcholine molecules which facilitate the transmission of nerve impulses from one nerve cell to another. The easier flow of messages within the nervous system may make it easier to retrieve them as well.

To say that time heals all wounds with respect to thoughts, is to say that the molecules representing the thoughts are decaying with time. We are less angry at someone today than we were last week because these thought molecules have undergone decay of some sort. It is tempting to suggest that the more we use our brain, the less molecular decay there is. If sensory input continues at a relatively high level over our entire lifetime, memory molecules continue to be made and will replace those that have been destroyed. This is not to say old age will not bring on memory loss, because some memories will fade, but new memories will be formed and will balance to some extent those lost. The mentally active older person has compensated for molecular destruction by molecular resynthesis. Pablo Casals, Pablo Picasso, Margaret Mead, George Bernard Shaw, and Agatha Christie are examples of people who aged really only in appearance, not in mental activity. These people do not prove the above speculation, since there may be an equal number of creative people who have aged badly. However, some recent research has shown that blood flow to parts of the brain increases with mental activity. It may be that continued mental activity throughout life helps to supply the brain's nerve cells with the proper nutrients via blood flow so that brain function is not too badly impaired with age.

DREAMS, CREATIVITY, AND INTUITION   We saw in chapter 2 that dreams may serve to combine new experiences with old ones and to lay down new memory patterns in a way that the awake brain might not be able to accomplish. Dreams are made up from what information we have in storage—that is, from memory. If the information is not in memory, we cannot dream about it. The stringing together of these memory molecules in some way may produce a thought, much in the same way that stringing together letters can produce a sentence. Sometimes in dreams, the memory molecules come together to produce a rather reasonable story. At other times, the molecules get together in unpredictable ways to produce a bizarre chain of events. During the dream stage of sleep there is less control in putting together memory-molecule sequences than in the wakeful state. We are creative in our dreams for this very reason.

Creativity can be defined as the putting together of old information in new ways. An invention, in these terms, is nothing more than taking what is known and assembling it in a new way. Crystals and wires existed before someone put them together to form a crystal radio set. Even something like the invention of the wheel would meet the definition of creativity. The first wheel may have been a circular slab of wood. Wood and circles existed, but putting them together in a new way to move something produced the wheel. Creativity in the arts involves putting together preexisting materials in a new way; creative writing is the putting together of old words in new ways. How our brains are creative in this way we do not know, but in terms of memory molecules, one could imagine that these molecules are associating with one another more readily in creative people. To be creative, there has to be something in memory first. The more information learned, the greater the number of memory molecules and the greater the chance they may combine to form new thoughts. If thinking involves the manipulation of stored information, then the more learning we have done, the better. This is, in fact, the basis of education, or at least its hope. But of course the key to creativity is having the "right" information stored (since most of what is stored may be useless) and then controlling the association of these memory molecules. Unfortunately, no one can say specifically what one needs to learn in order to be creative, and there is no way to control the association of memory molecules into creative thoughts. Each profession has its required curriculum, which generates a minimum number of memory molecules to start the practitioner thinking like a member of the profession. The rest is up to the individual or rather to his or her molecules. Even child prodigies do not assemble their creations out of whole cloth. Mozart apparently learned enough from his harpsichord lessons at three to be able to compose musical pieces at four. His extraordinary brain had the ability to associate a minimal amount of information in new ways. But not even such a person can create something with nothing in memory.

The suggestion here is that an element of chance

enters into creativity, because some thought combinations may result from a random stringing together of memory molecules. The single brilliant discovery or insight of a genius may well be produced by the chance assembly of his or her molecules into a unique thought. As we saw, this thought must be created out of past information already stored in memory and must then be recognized by the person as being of significance. Part of genius is the ability to recognize the importance of one's discovery. On the other hand, the genius who continues to produce one brilliant thing after another is not relying just on chance effects in his or her brain. As with Mozart, the molecules must be selected in some unknown way so as to be strung together in unique ways more often than chance would dictate, and certainly more often than happens to most of us.

Some people can work quite effectively, at times, using their intuition. They come to a good decision or develop an idea without being aware of how they got it. However, while the idea might seem to have appeared magically, there may be reason to suggest it actually is the result of information processing in the brain that we are not aware of. We saw earlier in the chapter that any given memory might be located in several places in the brain. Furthermore, it may be that some parts of the brain do not communicate with other parts the memories they have actually stored. Only when a thought has been constructed from the memories does another part of the brain know what has happened. A thought could appear seemingly out of nowhere to give us our feeling of intuition, when in fact it was produced from memory in a part of the brain where the information processing was going on without our awareness. Then the thought pops into our awareness, and not being aware of its development, we call it intuition.

DECISIONS, DECISIONS   What is stored in memory is also important to the process of decision making. Decision making involves choosing among alternatives. Do we do this or that? If we have a choice to make, that means we have stored alternative courses of action in memory. Some alternatives may have been recalled from previously stored information; others may recently have been placed in memory storage. For instance, in deciding what automobile route to take to a vacation spot, we might have several alternatives in memory: the auto club's suggested route, a friend's suggested route, and a route suggested by recent traffic information. Our brain in some way selects from among these alternatives, but we have no idea how this is accomplished at the molecular level. In view of the belief that we usually choose the best alternative consciously, it would be particularly interesting to know the extent to which molecules made our choice without our knowledge. One could imagine one of the alternatives randomly popping out of memory storage, rather than our selecting the molecules representing that alternative in memory. Perhaps bad decision makers are more prone to this than good decision makers! Thus bad decision makers exert less control over molecular events in the selection process. Once out, the molecular representation of the alternative is considered by us to be our best choice, when actually we do not know whether it was or not. We rationalize our choice by explaining it on the basis of having freely chosen among alternatives, when there may actually be another explanation.

A MOLECULAR SCENARIO OF DECISION MAKING

We have considered the possibility that thinking may result from either conscious choice or from random movements of molecules. Most of us are more comfortable with the notion that our thoughts are controlled by our will, which produces orderly decisions, but let us consider an example that will emphasize the random nature of thinking. Not all decision making may take place this way, but the example is worth considering. A woman has just moved to a new apartment. The wall behind her sofa is bare. Her long-term memory molecules remind her that the sofas she has seen have paintings hanging above them. The molecules that tell her everyone has such a painting produce the desire or motivation to get one. These molecules initiate nerve signals that would alert her to look for art galleries and activate her muscles to move her to them at the proper time. On the way to work one morning, she sees a painting in a gallery window. Of all the sights coming into her brain, a store that sells paintings is going to be of special interest because this particular visual pattern will be recognized as something to respond to. What she sees of the painting in driving by she likes, even though her visual sense is not at its rhythmic peak. This painting goes into short-term memory. After work, she drops by the gallery, but now with her visual sense at its peak, the painting does not look so good. The part of her brain that handles pictorial details rejects it. The molecules representing this painting break apart and the picture is forgotten. She is shown other paintings. Information about them goes into short-term memory molecules: their size, price, color, etc. She is about to make a decision, but she does not know it yet. Diverse thoughts about the painting are being constructed in her brain by the tying together of memory molecules about the painting. One painting has a better price, one is a better color for her room, one is a better size, another is a more appropriate style, and so on. From among the thoughts representing each painting, one will be selected to buy. By chance, one thought produces nerve signals that get to the language center of her brain first, and she says, "I'll take that one." The thoughts (strings of memory molecules) about the other paintings start to break apart in short-term memory, and the merits of these paintings fade away in comparison to the one selected, whose thought has entered long-term memory and relative preservation. She will say proudly to her friends, "I chose this one as the best." In fact, the choice was made randomly, and then even rationalized! Rationalization may be no more than the molecular decay of the thoughts of alternative action. Her free choice was an illusion. Is this an oversimplification? Maybe, maybe not.

OUR PLASTIC BRAIN   The fact that we can learn and remember indicates that our brain chemistry can be changed, and this is important because learning changes the way we look at the world by changing our patterns of thinking. We would like to know, though, just how malleable (plastic) our brain is. To what extent can it be shaped like warm plastic by external influences? It is generally acknowledged that our genes set limits on our behavior, but our surroundings and our motivation determine how widely we range. We may be born athletically gifted, yet may not choose to pursue sports or may not get proper coaching or facilities to reach our potential. We know the molecular intricacies of thinking have to be determined at least in part by our genes, or the appropriate cells in the human embryo would not be directed to form the brain during development. The way the brain is put together in turn determines how the brain functions and how we think. But our genes cannot do it all, and that is why we can acquire memory of the things around us. I pointed out that memory may reside in the connections among brain nerve cells. There may be a total of one thousand trillion of these connections in our brain, but we may have no more than half a million different genes in our body. Therefore, our genes cannot possibly be responsible for producing all these connections because there are not enough genes. What may well produce these connections is input from our surroundings, which produces memory.

The impact of our environment upon our molecules may produce changes in our brain that we have not planned on. We often learn something without trying to, and this may be just as important as what we try to learn. If what we learn is unplanned, our thinking may be influenced in ways we are not aware of. Experiments with newborn rats raised in an enriched environment that gave them plenty of playthings and playmates showed that these rats developed different brains than those raised in an impoverished environment, isolated from each other and lacking playthings such as ladders and tunnels. The brains of the enriched rats showed an increase in size in some brain areas and a change in brain chemistry. As humans age, we expect some brain nerve cells to die off, but as it turns out, some nerve cells also show an increase in the complexity of their structure, even up to age eighty or so. Living this long gives us more time to capture the environment into our brain molecules. Experiments with kittens raised in an environment consisting only of vertical stripes in their line of vision showed that these kittens' brain cells would later only respond to those stripes and not to horizontal ones. Similarly, if raised under horizontal-stripe conditions, vertical stripes would not be recognized by the kittens.

These kinds of experiments indicate that the environment can affect the development of the brain's structure and function. If such plastic changes are also widespread in humans, then some of our subsequent reactions to the world would be programmed in at an early age. Of course psychologists have been saying this for years, but now the biological evidence is beginning to come in from the laboratories. Would it not be fascinating if early exposure to classical music predisposed our brain cells and their molecules to respond more positively in later life to classical than to popular music? For example, early exposure to classical music may produce in the musical side of our brain memory molecules that encode information about such things as rhythmic patterns and melodic lines. These memory molecules are strung together to produce thoughts about what kind of music sounds pleasant, that is, familiar. As we listen to more music, information about other kinds of music would also enter memory storage. Thoughts about this music would not meet the standards of pleasure set up in memory by classical music, so classical music would be preferred. Could early exposure to certain types of paintings direct our brain cells to be more attentive to certain patterns of color and shape? There is no end to what we can imagine as having a permanent effect upon our brain and behavior, an effect totally unanticipated.

MOTIVATION   The desire to act and to do something is what we call motivation. We know that when motivated, we behave differently than when not, because motivation activates behavior. If motivated, we can perform better, whether what is involved is thinking or learning, working or playing. We have seen that behavior is not independent of what molecules are doing in our body; motivation offers yet another example of this. Something within us determines whether we wish to get up off our bottoms and accomplish something. Call it free will or ambition if you must, but whatever it is, it has a great influence upon our behavior. No one doubts this motivating effect upon our behavior, but we cannot point specifically to what determines how badly we want something. In molecular terms, motivation may speed up the recall of memory molecules and accelerate their assembly into thoughts, which are then translated into action. To say we are motivated to do something may be to say that chemicals are released in our brain that allow memory molecules to be linked together to form thoughts of action. Those with high motivational levels may well have brains where the release of these chemicals is much more frequent than it is in people with low motivational levels.

We have ever-varying desires to engage in a variety of behaviors such as eating, drinking, playing, working, and sexual activity. We know that external events such as rewards can influence the initiation of these behaviors. Money, power, and pleasure are powerful motivators, but within limits, our behavior is driven internally to seek what our molecules do not have. It is as though there is a reference point determined by a configuration of molecules which, when deviated from, activates a behavior that will return us to the reference point. Something like this motivates us to eat when hungry, to drink when thirsty, and to stop after certain levels of intake. These are examples of the individual deviating from and returning to the internal reference point.

Even more interesting examples develop when the internal reference point changes. If our internal body temperature is lowered, experiments have shown that a cool stimulus placed on our skin is considered unpleasant, while a warm stimulus is considered pleasant. However, when our internal body temperature is raised, the same cool stimulus now becomes pleasant and the same warm stimulus becomes unpleasant. Therefore, the internal state (temperature, in this case) of our body determines how a stimulus is perceived. In chapter 2 we saw another example of this, except there the perception of sights, sounds, and smells was influenced by internal circadian rhythms in our senses. The temperature experiments demonstrate that the same external stimulus will be perceived differently if the internal state of the organism changes. In this case, the motivation would be to avoid certain unpleasant temperatures and approach pleasant ones. This conclusion is supported by another experiment in which people who had fasted were given about four tablespoons of a sugar solution every three minutes or so. It tasted very pleasant over the first thirty minutes, but gradually became very unpleasant by seventy minutes. The reason for this change was that the number of blood-sugar molecules was increasing. As they reached a maximum level, they caused the body to respond unpleasantly to sugar in the mouth in order to prevent more sugar from entering the body. Again, the internal reference point (blood-sugar level, in this case) changed, as did our behavior in response to a constant external stimulus (the sugar solution). The motivation not to drink more of the sugar solution was determined by the internal state of our molecules. If our motivation to do a variety of other things is as much internally directed as these simple examples, one wonders who is controlling whom.

OUR DIVIDED BRAIN AND GENIUSES   The problem of behavior control also arises between the two hemispheres or halves of our brain. The halves of the brain look slightly different from each other, and they perform some functions that are different, indicating that one side will exert control over certain functions. The dominant side of the brain for right-handed people is the left; it is particularly adapted to language and arithmetic skills and the analysis of detail. In contrast, the right side handles musical, pictorial, and pattern-recognition skills better. For left-handers, the dominant side for language could be the right or the left. Each side can handle the other's functions, but for these behaviors, not nearly as well. These findings have come mostly from observing people who have had one of their hemispheres injured or operated on, with a resultant deficit in one or more of these skills. Even more distinctions between the two sides of the brain are likely to be found in the future.

It is well known (which means I have not bothered to look up the exact date of discovery) that different anatomical sites in the brain deal with different parts of the body, such as receiving information from the senses or controlling limb movement. However, the finding of very highly specialized areas to deal with specific complex mental processes is relatively new. These behaviors depend, then, on quite specific pieces of brain tissue (and their underlying molecular structure) to process relevant information. The ability to read notes of music, for instance, and translate them into the appropriate movement of the hands and feet or mouth (eye-limb coordination) would depend initially upon the extent of development of the musical center of our right brain hemisphere, as well as upon muscular coordination centers in other parts of the brain. Practice serves to put together memory molecules of a musical nature for processing by these centers. However, if the brain cells of the musical center are not specialized enough to handle molecules encoding musical information, our musical ability will be slight. A gifted composer would result, as we saw earlier in this chapter, if the manipulation of the appropriate memory molecules by the music center produced unique combinations of sounds. Similarly, a mathematically gifted person would have a well-developed left side of the brain, as would someone with a gift for languages. You either have it or you don't—the molecules decide.

Regardless of which side of the brain we are talking about, it is interesting to speculate why there are musical and mathematical geniuses at a young age. These child prodigies do not appear in the fields of history, sociology, literature, or art, for example. The reason for this may be that these fields do not have the same logical structures to them as mathematics and music. These particular logical structures seem somehow to be duplicated in the brain wiring of those who can do mathematics or compose and play music with considerable skill. Certain parts of their brain developed, quite by chance, into structures that function according to the same rules governing how mathematics and music are created. That is, the logic of the brain language used to process information in these brain centers mirrors the logic of the language of music and mathematics.

INTELLIGENCE   There are any number of IQ (intelligence quotient) tests that purport to measure intelligence, but how can we be sure that intelligence is being measured? IQ tests only measure IQ because intelligence has not been defined in biological terms. We can go further, as some have, and even say that intelligence never existed as a concept until it was measured. It is an artifact of psychological testing. The concept of intelligence may have no real meaning, no real basis in the molecular reality of the brain. IQ tests attempt to measure brain function without actually looking inside the brain. Herein lies the problem with psychology, which too often regards us as a box to probe and prod but not to look into. Biologists, in contrast, rip it open. If you do not look inside something you cannot figure out how it works. As an analogy you can ask a computer to do all sorts of things for you, and measure what it does, but it will tell you nothing about how a computer works. You will learn nothing of binary codes and integrated electronic circuits, the stuff of computers. You have to look inside to find them. IQ tests, and in fact all psychological tests, measure a limited output of our brain as determined by how we answer certain questions. This output (our answers) is said to correlate well with our intelligence, but unfortunately "things are not correlated in nature." Either IQ tests measure intelligence or they do not.

IQ tests are useful in assessing such things as brain damage, for after all, if our brain is damaged, its output will be altered and such tests will pick this up. IQ tests also predict with some success how well a child will do in school. But these assessments are not without difficulties, and the main one has to do with cultural bias. People in any culture who develop and use IQ tests are already assuming intelligence is worth measuring (the cultural bias is that someone should take an IQ test), and they tie the measurement of intelligence to the prevalent educational philosophy. Therefore, if you do not know what the culture thinks you should know (or do not reason the same way it does), then you cannot, by the definition of the intelligence test, be intelligent. The Soviets have made effective use of this logic. If the Soviets think they have created the best of all existing worlds, then anyone who does not like this world is certainly not intelligent—possibly even mentally ill—and needs reeducation, and retraining.

The point about intelligence is this: We do not know how to measure it directly because it is not a single entity. Intelligence really is the sum total of an untold number of molecular events—ranging from how well our senses code environmental information; through decision-making ability, creativity, and motivation; to the manipulation of molecules into thought. To say that an IQ test of a handful of questions can measure all this accurately is to fool ourselves. It surely measures a part of this, but far from all of it.

NEARSIGHTEDNESS AND INTELLIGENCE   There is some evidence that nearsightedness has a genetic basis and is not due to excessive amounts of reading and poor lighting conditions. Twin studies have shown that identical twin pairs are more likely to be nearsighted than fraternal twin pairs if one twin is nearsighted. Some have speculated that the genes for "intelligence" may also affect the development of the eyes in such a way that nearsightedness results. For what it is worth, IQ scores tend to be significantly higher for the nearsighted. Of course, not all those who wear glasses are more intelligent; some just cannot see well. Do those who cannot see well because of their nearsightedness stay inside and read and increase their chances of scoring well on IQ tests? Probably not, since it has been shown that some people scoring high on

IQ tests as young children do not develop nearsightedness until the teenage years.

One could imagine that hundreds of thousands of years ago these humans or near-humans who were nearsighted were more likely to be eaten by animals they could not see approaching, or were more likely to fall off a cliff, etc. Since the nearsighted would be less likely to survive and reproduce, they would have fewer children who would pass the nearsightedness-intelligence genes on. Much more recently, as living became less harsh and as glasses for the nearsighted became available, the incidence of nearsightedness would increase, since these people would then have a better chance than before of living long enough to reproduce and pass their nearsightedness genes on. All things being equal, more intelligent people should be around—but where are they?

FACIAL EXPRESSIONS   Whatever intelligence is, or is not, most of us still have a notion about who looks intelligent and who does not. Whether we could agree on what it takes to look intelligent, I do not know, but certainly some of it has to do with how the person is dressed. We have learned to expect in Western society that a man or woman dressed in a business suit and carrying a briefcase is going to be more intelligent than someone in faded pants and a sloppy shirt. But strip them of their clothes and see who looks more intelligent. Without their trappings we might not be able to agree on who looks intelligent and who does not. On the other hand, maybe those who are intelligent really look intelligent and those who are stupid look stupid. I know this is going to sound like phrenology (the nineteenth-century false belief that mental abilities could be measured by the shape of the skull), but perhaps the same molecular events that shape the brain processes involved in intelligence also shape the face and its expressions. In the extreme this is true, for those with Down's syndrome (mongolism) have slanted eyes, a flattened nose bridge, an opened mouth, and a relatively short head—all coupled with a very low IQ. We associate their looks with their low intelligence. Perhaps there is an intelligent look and a stupid look that do reflect brain capabilities.

On much more solid ground, we can say that there are facial expressions which at least reflect underlying emotions. At birth the human infant has all the working facial muscles necessary to produce a variety of expressions similar to those adults use. Newborns, for instance, will show a "disgust" expression when presented with an unpleasant taste. The expressions for happiness, anger, sadness, disgust, and a fear-surprise combination seem to be universal. They are found in all peoples throughout the world. The fact that some of these are also found in children born both deaf and blind suggests these basic facial expressions are not merely learned, but are present from birth. After all, it is impossible to imagine how one both deaf and blind could learn these expressions by watching or hearing others.

When confronted with a situation that produces one of these responses, such as surprise, we do not stop to think what facial expression to produce. Instead, it is produced spontaneously; it is a natural reaction. The molecular events producing these feelings within the brain are signaled by facial expressions to communicate our feelings to others. This allows other people to react accordingly. No doubt this form of communication evolved before spoken language did, because it is a more simple behavior.

THINKING ABOUT MOVEMENT   While the muscular movements in facial expressions are pretty much automatic, we might ask how we initiate voluntary muscular movements. Such muscular movements are necessary for us to write with our fingers, to gesture with our hands, or to move from one place to another with our legs. Before the muscles which produce these movements actually start to move, they must receive nerve signals from the brain. We initiate these impulses by thinking about movement. Somehow we "will" atoms and molecules to move across nerve-cell membranes to start a nerve signal in an appropriate part of the brain. The signal is then transmitted to muscles to produce movement. Suppose you want to raise your arm—you can do it anytime you want to. You do it by directing your atoms and molecules to move! How we start the molecules rolling is not known. It takes a thought to do it, but what generates the thought? Thinking about thinking is difficult because we are asking the brain to examine itself.

THINKING ABOUT TIME   In dreaming, our sense of time is often distorted, mixing together past and present happenings. Sometimes in dreams we are not aware of time passing, and a long series of events passes by very quickly. While awake the same thing often happens, and time passes at different speeds according to what we are doing and what is happening to us. We saw in chapter 2 that we have a rhythm in body temperature. Well, there is also a rhythm in time perception that follows the temperature rhythm.

As our internal body temperature increases—not only as part of our temperature rhythm, but also if we have a fever—time seems to speed up. As our internal body temperature decreases in its circadian rhythm, time seems to slow down. Since our sense of time varies with our temperature, it is reasonable to suppose that the more our molecules in our brain move around, the faster time appears to pass. The less they move around, the slower time appears to pass. When we are bored and time seems to pass slowly, it is because we are not getting enough stimulation from our surroundings. Not much stimulation means our senses are not converting our surroundings to molecular events. Consequently, there is relatively not much molecular movement. Conversely, when we are having a great time because we are stimulated by what is around us, then our senses are very active and produce a great deal of molecular movement. If we spend one hour enjoying ourselves, and it seems like three hours have passed, then time *appears* to have speeded up. In reality time passed more slowly than we thought, as only one hour passed, not three hours. I am concerned with only what *appears* to have happened to time.

What molecules are involved in time perception is not known, but we know that certain drug molecules can interact with these time molecules to affect our sense of time. For some people marijuana speeds up their sense of time and tranquilizers make time pass more slowly. Tranquilizers slow up nerve impulses and therefore relax us. Marijuana speeds up some nerve impulses so that we have heightened awareness of our surroundings, even though its overall effect is to relax us. Apparently some of the molecules affected by both marijuana and tranquilizers are the ones involved in our sense of time. These drugs are not affecting molecules all throughout our body, but rather at certain of the connections between our nerve cells. It is here that our sense of time originates.

DÉJÀ VU   Déjà vu is a phenomenon we all experience at one time or another. It is the "I-have-seen-it-before-but-I-couldn't-have" trick that our memory plays on us. If we walk into a room that we have never been in before, or visit a place for the first time, and feel it looks all too familiar, then we are experiencing déjà vu. In these instances, certain features of what we see correspond to similar features that have already been stored in long-term memory from some previous experience or even from a dream. Our brain is picking out and recognizing just *some* specific familiar features of our new surroundings, but reacts as though the *entire* new surroundings are familiar. In other words, we see something in a new situation that is similar to something we have previously experienced and which is stored in memory. Our brain interprets this as having seen the whole thing before. The more we have stored in long-term memory (the more we read, see, experience, etc.), the more likely it would seem for déjà vu to occur. Any time our brain fools us, we can suspect we are not in total control of ourselves. We are, of course, also fooled by optical illusions where, say, two lines of equal length are judged to be unequal in length. This is a consequence of the way in which the visual center of our brain processes information.

MALE-FEMALE BRAIN DIFFERENCES Throughout this chapter it has been assumed that there is no difference between human male and female brains. This assumption is not correct in certain instances. Human male brains on the average are about eleven percent larger than female brains, but this probably represents just an overall body-size difference. Whales and elephants, for example, have brains more than twice as large as human brains. The hypothalamus and pituitary parts of the brain are chemically different between males and females. The hypothalamus causes the release of a variety of hormones from the pituitary; these hormones may not only be released at different times for men and women, but different hormones may be involved as well. For example, after women give birth, a hormone (oxytocin) is released by the brain that leads to contraction of the uterus and facilitates ejection of milk from the breasts. Other hormones are, of course, released under brain control to produce the menstrual cycle. For men, the hypothalamus and pituitary release hormones to stimulate sperm production.

These differences between human male and female brains are quite real and are easily measured. Even more differences between male and female brains have been found in animals. In rats and hamsters, differences in the pattern of nerve connections between males and females can be seen under a microscope. The differences are caused by sex hormones early in life. Castrating newborn male rats leads to the development of femalelike nerve connections; giving newborn female rats the male hormone testosterone leads to the development of male-like nerve connections.

With all the documented male-female brain differences, one begins to suspect that there are certainly more of them to be discovered. Can one now begin to say that some of the observed differences in behavior between human males and females have their origin in the molecules of the brain? Some of the ways males and females differ from each other in their behavior are clearly learned. Women behave differently in the way they dress, using lipstick and eye shadow, for example. Boys play with guns, girls play with dolls; men learn to play football, women do not; and so on. But there are differences in some more fundamental behaviors that may not be learned. It is well known that on the average, females have greater language skills and verbal ability than males do, while males have greater spatial, visual, and mathematical skills. This is a general statement—clearly there are exceptions in behavior for both sexes. These differences become particularly noticeable by the age of thirteen or fourteen. No doubt part of the reason for these skill differences is the way boys and girls are treated in Western societies. If girls are expected to do better in English classes and boys to do better in math classes, then each sex will be pushed by parents, teachers, and fellow students to do better in what is expected of them. However, the major reason for these skill differences may be that the organization of the brain is slightly different for males and females. It follows then that by and large the great painters of the past should have been men because men excel in visual skills. By the same reasoning, most of the great writers of the past should have been women because of their verbal and language skills. Not so, however, because in the past women had little or no opportunities to acquire training and education. Their molecular advantage could not be expressed.

One evolutionary reason for these skill differences would be that men were the hunters (because they were stronger or because they did not have to nurse infants?) and only those with the best visual skills could kill animals to eat. Those with lesser visual skills could not survive, because they did not kill enough to eat or in turn were eaten by what they were hunting. As our species was evolving, men and women could have had equal visual skills, but if women were not out hunting, there would have been no selection process that weeded out those who saw less well. Consequently for the population as a whole, women's visual skills were unchanged, but men's visual skills were improving on the average because those who saw less well were no longer around. We could also propose that language skills were the same for men and women. For women organizing child care and food gathering and preparation, language skills became very important. Those women who could not adequately communicate their needs may have been at a disadvantage, not receiving the care and cooperation they needed to survive. Hence for the female population as a whole, women's language skills were improving compared to men's. Hunting for the men may have required no language skills, particularly if they hunted alone.

The male edge in mathematical skills, it is said, may be a consequence of his visual skills and the females' language skills. Mathematics is symbol manipulation, and man's alleged visual-skill advantage may allow him to deal more easily with these visual symbols. Women, on the other hand, may tend to deal with mathematical symbols verbally rather than as visual objects, and something is lost in the translation process. We were not there when these differences might have emerged, so we cannot say what really happened, but it is fun to guess. The important point in all this is that there may be biological reasons, as well as the environmental ones, for some important male-female behavior differences. If so, we cannot fail to be impressed once again that our molecules are setting the stage for what we can and cannot do.

THE FUTURE OF THINKING   If we can sort out all the kinds of molecules involved in all the facets of our thinking processes, then we can change the way we think. We can develop memory-improvement pills to get our memory molecules out of storage, and dream pills to call out from our thoughts and into our dreams those molecules that represent the most triumphant personal moments imagined. Why not forgetting pills for those bad memories? These would be chemicals that break up selected memory molecules. We could take pills to motivate us and pills to release lots of memory molecules to combine into new thoughts to make us more creative. We could take pills to speed up our sense of time when what we are doing is boring and pills to slow up our sense of time when we wish to prolong the enjoyable moments. We could improve our skills by taking memory pills that would put into our brain the necessary memory molecules to give us a new foreign language, a history of the ancient world, or a knowledge of algebra. It could be as easy as slipping a new cassette into the old tape deck.

I doubt that we will see anything quite this good (or bad) in our lifetime, as we know so little now. Nevertheless, the potential for these kinds of treatments is here, and it would change the way we do things. If we could put information directly into our memory we would have to redesign much of our educational system, which depends a great deal on getting facts through our thick skulls. If we could directly read out what is in a person's memory we would have to redesign our court-trial systems where plaintiffs, defendants, and witnesses are questioned by lawyers and judges to find out what is in their memories. But then if we could read *out* their memories, someone could read *in* other ones just as well. Bribery of witnesses and jurors would be transformed to directly altering memory molecules. The truth may always be elusive.

Thinking has often been considered to be some mysterious process functioning somehow apart from the physiology of the body. This chapter has presented evidence to the contrary by emphasizing the chemical nature of thinking. Like all the behaviors discussed so far, thinking has a molecular basis. Someday we will even be able to talk about the molecules involved in such thoughts as hope, despair, guilt, trust, pity, and indignation. But for now we must wait.

4

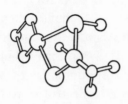

Molecular Madness

When something goes wrong with our thinking processes, regardless of the reasons, we can be considered mentally ill in a general sense, just as when something goes wrong with our bodily physiology we are considered physically ill. It is not always clear just how distorted our thinking has to be before we are considered mentally ill. There are no lab tests to establish mental disorders the way there are to establish the presence of diabetes or anemia, so diagnosis relies fundamentally on subjective opinions. Because of this, there is often disagreement among people dealing with the mentally ill as to who is ill, what to call it, and how to treat it. As the psychiatrist Thomas Szasz said, "If you talk to God, you are praying. . . . If God talks to you, you have schizophrenia."

An example of the problem is illustrated by an experiment that was conducted in 1973 in twelve mental-health hospitals on the East and West coasts by eight sane-regular-normal-average people. These people showed how easily a misdiagnosis in psychiatry can occur. Separately, they called a hospital for an appointment. Upon arrival they complained of having heard voices, but once admitted to the hospitals they acted normal and displayed no abnormal symptoms whatsoever. In all but one case, these pseudopatients (as they were called) were diagnosed as schizophrenic and were treated accordingly by the hospital staffs during their stays. For example, one pseudopatient paced the halls because he was bored, but a nurse asked him if he was nervous, assuming something was wrong with him. Another pseudopatient wrote notes about his experiences in the hospital, and did it often and in view of the staff. No one looked at what he wrote or asked him about it. His continued writing was considered to be a result of his disturbance. Nobody in his right mind writes all the time! Nevertheless, after an average stay of nineteen days, the pseudopatients convinced the staff by their behavior that they "exhibited no abnormal indications," and were released. But they were not released free from mental illness as far as their medical records were concerned. They were released as schizophrenics in remission—showing relief from schizophrenia, but schizophrenics nonetheless. They were sane people, but a label was put on them, and it stuck throughout their hospital stay, even though they behaved perfectly normally. In some cases, distinguishing the sane from the insane is not always easily done, as this experiment has shown.

An implication of this study is that the social environment we find ourselves in determines how others look at us. We may all get a good deal of attention at our offices, particularly if we are the bosses, but when we go somewhere else where we are unknown, no one treats us specially. The pseudopatients were in a mental institution and hence were considered by the staff to be mentally ill. This raises the question of whether mental illness in fact exists in any absolute sense, or whether it is always relative to other people's expectations of behavior. If we behave differently from most people, are we considered mentally ill simply because we do not behave as expected? Do the same kinds of mentally ill behaviors occur throughout the world in a variety of cultural environments (the absolute viewpoint) or do they depend upon what cultures they are found in (the relative viewpoint)? If abnormal behavior in one culture is considered normal in another, then the relative viewpoint is supported, because how well you are considered to be is relative to what others think is normal. As is usually the case in a complex, little-understood area like mental illness, there is also support for the opposite viewpoint. A 1976 study reported that members of two quite distinct non-Western cultures (Alaskan Eskimos and Nigerian Yorubas) exhibited the same type of schizo-phrenialike behavior as is found in Western cultures. Not only do the behavioral aberrations of schizophrenics seem to be similar throughout the world, but also the incidence of schizophrenia throughout Europe, Asia, and the United States is about the same (0.3 percent of the population). One conclusion to draw from both the relative and absolute viewpoints is that mental illness is a real sickness found throughout the world, but its diagnosis is influenced in one way or another by the beliefs of those doing the diagnosing. Therefore, while a person may be mentally ill, there will not always be agreement on what to call it. Psychiatrists trained in different countries (or even at different schools within the same country) may call the same behavior by different names. There are diagnostic guides to follow, but interpretation of them is still a personal matter.

MOLECULAR MADNESS   If someone is mentally ill, something is wrong somewhere in the molecules of the brain. It is as simple as that, and as complicated as that. There are no gross anatomical defects revealed at autopsy in the brains of the mentally ill—although using the newly developed computer-assisted X-ray scans known as CAT scans (computerized axial tomography) of the brain, structural differences are starting to show up between schizophrenics and nonschizophrenics. The madness is molecular and therefore more subtle, more difficult to detect and to comprehend. Any number of things could be going wrong. Each of our brain cells contains about ten billion molecules of proteins, vitamins, fats, carbohydrates, nucleic acids (DNA and related chemicals), and their component parts. These molecules are the cell; they give it a highly organized structure and perform its functions. Being composed of such an enormous number of parts that must work in harmony to prevent chaos, a cell is easily harmed. X rays, heat, cold, pollutants in our air, and water and chemicals in our food have all been shown to cause damage to our cells. Lead and mercury poisoning are known to affect our nervous system. We may also be born with cells that do not function quite properly because of errors in the cells' genes. We know that there are over two dozen genetic diseases (defects in the DNA) that produce severe mental retardation. In short, a cell can be harmed by just about anything if it is present in a high enough concentration ("the poison is in the dose") or if the concentration of chemicals that compose the cell is lowered. Too little vitamin A, for instance, causes dryness of the skin, while too much causes a skin rash to develop.

There is reason to suspect that some forms of mental illness are produced by improper concentrations of molecules within certain regions of the brain. In a disease called PKU (phenylketonuria), the enzyme is defective that facilitates the molecular conversion in cells of the amino acid phenylalanine to another type of amino acid called tyrosine. Consequently, phenylalanine piles up and gets converted by other enzymes into a variety of other molecules not normally present in such concentrations. The result is mental illness in the form of mental retardation. If treatment is started soon enough after birth, when the disease can be detected, elimination of phenylalanine from the diet stops the disease and prevents mental retardation.

People deficient in vitamin B_1 (thiamine) show mental confusion; those deficient in vitamin B_3 (niacin) show mental deterioration, among other things. Providing adequate concentrations of these vitamins eliminates the problems, and vitamin B_1 deficiency (beriberi) and B_3 deficiency (pellagra) are not much heard of in the United States. A test for PKU in newborns is done routinely in most hospitals so that early diagnosis and treatment are possible. Molecular psychiatry can restore the concentrations of three types of molecules (phenylalanine, vitamins B_1 and B_3) to normal levels and all but eliminate these kinds of mental illnesses in America. It is important to note, however, that the occasional sufferer of these diseases is not now said to be suffering from some vague thing called mental illness. The cause of the illness has been ascertained and it is called PKU or a vitamin B_1 or B_3 deficiency.

Similarly, the delusions, hallucinations, and depression that can accompany the last stage of a syphilis infection are now called brain disorders. Syphilis is caused by a bacterial infection obtained not from toilet seats. Many years after the initial infection, if untreated, the bacteria invade the nervous system and eventually may produce the mental disturbances. Penicillin cures the disease in the early stages by destroying the bacteria and preventing subsequent mental disorders. Any number of non-nervous system infections by microorganisms that produce a high fever—such as malaria, typhoid fever, pneumonia, and typhus—can also produce impairment of intellectual function, leading to delirium. Those affected act confused, perplexed, vague, disoriented, and generally "out of it." Actual infection of the brain itself, as in bacterial meningitis and viral encephalitis, can also produce delirium. When most of the adrenal glands (located over the kidneys) are destroyed by Addison's disease, the afflicted may become seriously depressed, irritable, and paranoid. Treatment with chemicals isolated from healthy adrenals eliminates the mental problems. In New England, when the United States was being settled, the Devil was thought to possess those who exhibited jerking motions, rage, and intellectual deterioration. We now know these behaviors resulted from Huntington's chorea, a relatively rare metabolic disease of the nervous system. Some tumors of the brain can also produce severe mental disorders. These are but a few of the known causes of mental illness of one sort or another. Since we know the causes of these mental illnesses, we do not call them mental illness any more!

One begins to wonder if many of the mental illnesses we now call schizophrenia, paranoia, and depression, to name a few, will someday also be removed from the mental-illness category as the above disorders have been, and more appropriately be called metabolic, genetic, or deficiency diseases or brain disorders. For a long time, problems with our thinking processes have been called mental illness, until we could be more specific and call them something else. As we learn more, the division of illness into either physical or mental categories makes less and less sense, as one by one the mental illnesses fall into the physical pot. The move to the molecular or chemical and physical viewpoint is illustrated by the direction the sciences are taking. The study of psychology has become more like biology; biology has become more like chemistry; and chemistry is becoming more like physics. Maybe we should all study physics because it offers the most basic explanations.

Most importantly, these examples of mental illness I have mentioned were not caused by faulty interpersonal relationships, society's ills, sexual identity problems, unhappy childhoods, or traumatic life events. They were caused by microorganisms and metabolic molecular disorders, and we do not have to guess at what caused them anymore. There is nothing wrong with guessing, as it is a first approximation to the truth. But the more we learn, the less we have to guess.

CHEMICAL VERSUS PSYCHOLOGICAL CAUSES OF BEHAVIOR A chemical cause of behavior is synonymous with what is also called a neurological, organic, genetic, or physical cause of behavior. A psychological cause of behavior is called a psychosocial, learned, environmental, or psychiatric cause of behavior. We began to see in chapter 1, however, that a distinction between chemical and psychological causes is artificial: Psychological events can only affect our thinking and cause a behavior change through our senses, which convert all outside events to internal chemical events. If a mental illness does not have a chemical basis, it does not exist. It is not that a psychological approach to mental illness has no importance; rather it must be redefined in chemical terms. When people say someone has a psychological problem, they mean the problem is in the mind and not the body. But it's the same thing!—therefore a psychological problem is a real problem.

We can use male impotence (in the presence of a willing female) as an example to illustrate the traditional way a "physical" cause of a problem is distinguished from a "psychological" cause. When a man cannot produce an erection when he needs one, he is called impotent. Is this a physical or psychological problem? In common terms, is something wrong with his plumbing or his mind? Virtually all men have an erection every night during sleep. If a man suffering from impotence does not have erections during sleep, then all would agree he has a physical problem, such as an abnormal blood circulation to that polite area known as the groin. If he has an erection during sleep, then it is said it is only his mind holding him down when he is awake. Yet both the physical and psychological causes are producing molecular changes leading to impotence—so they are the same in this sense. Even better, recent research suggests that many cases of impotence are due to low levels of the male hormone testosterone. Injections of testosterone will straighten their impotence right out. The distress, anxiety, and depression that accompany impotence are probably the result and not the cause of the problem. If the right hormone molecules are not in the bloodstream heading for the groin because the brain does not release them under erotic stimulation, then an erection will not be possible. The chemistry of the brain and the body are involved together—there is no physical versus psychological distinction.

SCHIZOPHRENIA   Unfortunately, we are still guessing about the cause of schizophrenia, a mental disorder (or group of disorders) that has been known, some think, for the last three thousand years. Because we know so much more about it than about other mental illnesses, we can use it as a model for discussing the basic issues in all of molecular psychiatry. The schizophrenic exhibits hallucinations (sensing things when they in fact are not present), delusions (false beliefs), incoherent speech, and indifferent or hostile reactions to others. Schizophrenia is diagnosed if most of these behaviors are present and if chemical causes and infections like those mentioned can be ruled out. If we do not know for sure what caused these behaviors, then we call the behaviors schizophrenia —certainly not the best logic to follow. Consequently, many explanations have been offered about its causes and, as might be expected, they fall into two main categories: the chemical and the psychological (the same, right?).

One of the most popular psychological explanations of schizophrenia is that it is caused by emotional stress. The loss of someone near and dear, the inability to meet parental standards of behavior, and the inability to cope with life's constant demands are stress factors that many say will lead to schizophrenia. These are stresses common to most of us, but most of us do not become schizophrenic; only about 0.3 percent of us do. Most schizophrenia starts in late adolescence; it seldom begins after sixty years of age. Adolescence is certainly a time of stress in making the transition from child to adult, but it is also the time of significant hormone changes in the body as well. So stress is not the only influence on adolescents. The lower socioeconomic levels of society have the highest rates of schizophrenia, reflecting, some say, the increased stress of life found there. Others argue that the development of schizophrenia drives the person downward through society to the lower socioeconomic levels. After all, exhibiting the bizarre behavior of schizophrenia is not going to lead to invitations to become commodore of the local yacht club. In addition, even if schizophrenics do not drift into the lower levels of society—i.e., they were there to begin with—there is less good health care and nutrition there, which may serve to worsen the problem.

A brain virus infection or lack of proper vitamin levels would be equally good guesses as to what causes schizophrenia as stress is. Viruses have been found in the cerebrospinal fluid of schizophrenics, but as they can also be found in normal individuals this does not constitute proof of causation. Specific schizophrenic-inducing viruses would have to be found. A number of slow-acting viruses are known to affect the human central nervous system (the brain and spinal cord), taking many years to exert their effects. Some of these diseases, though rare, do cause mental deterioration. As we learn more about these viruses, we may find that they are much more common and relevant to the problem of mental illness. Vitamin deficits in the brain may cause mental illness. Vitamins are found in minute amounts in all cells, where their function is primarily to help enzymes work properly by actually combining with the molecular structure of the enzyme. If the proper number of vitamin molecules is not available, enzymes cannot function and certain required cellular processes will not continue. If these stopped processes relate to brain function, then mental illness could result. The human body cannot synthesize all its vitamin needs, so if the vitamins do not come into the body, there will be a problem. This is not meant to suggest that merely taking vitamin pills will cure mental illness, for there is no guarantee that the added vitamins will reach the appropriate brain cells. The body may destroy the vitamins before they get there. Also, the brain cells with the vitamin deficits may have been injured because of the deficits and be unable to take in vitamins through their cellular membranes.

Large urban centers have a larger proportion of schizophrenics—because there is more stress in large cities? Possibly, but schizophrenics may be attracted to large cities for better treatment facilities or to escape the talk and stares they elicit in small towns. Schizophrenia is found more often in females than in males, but it has not been demonstrated that women are subject to more stress then men, nor that women respond to stress less well than men do. However, divorced or separated women have a higher incidence of this illness than do married women. It is not clear whether the stress of marital difficulties helps to produce schizophrenia, or whether their schizophrenia caused their marital difficulties. Stress does have an impact upon our behavior (discussed in chapter 6), but to say that it alone causes schizophrenia is an unproven assumption. The only way to establish whether stress causes schizophrenia is to subject people to it and see if they become schizophrenic. This is the only way to prove if any part of our psychological and social environment causes mental illness, but it is not an ethical form of experimentation, so we do not have any proof of this kind.

Using a sample of a large number of people, one might be able to show that those people subjected to certain stress levels in their lives were more likely to become schizophrenic than similar people not reaching these stress levels. Finding such a relationship, though, does not prove that one causes the other. Any number of other things could be related to schizophrenia (and in fact could have caused it) but they were not measured!

Genes and Schizophrenia • The evidence is much better for a genetic basis of schizophrenia. This means a gene (or genes) for the behavior is inherited from the parents, although—as with any gene—its presence does not guarantee the behavior will occur, since the gene has to be turned on. It may be turned on by events in our environment or by events originating from inside the body. The absence of a gene, though, assures the behavior will not be present. Quite simply, we cannot fly unaided as a bird does, because we are not built like a bird—we do not have the genes that would give our body the structures to enable us to fly.

It could be that the stress put on a person turns on the genes for schizophrenia—we really do not know—but the support for stress, as discussed above, is not terribly compelling. This does not rule out the possibility of other environmental events turning on schizophrenic genes. For example, if one identical twin is schizophrenic, the other twin is far more likely to be schizophrenic than would be the case if they were fraternal twins. Identical twins arise from the union of one egg and one sperm. They are molecularly much closer to each other than fraternal twins, which arise from the union of two eggs with two sperms, and genetically are no more alike than children born at different times to the same mother and father. But if one identical twin is schizophrenic, the other twin is not always schizophrenic. This being so, the environment must play a role in turning on one twin's genes and not the other's, because it is assumed that identical twins have identical genes. There is no evidence, though, that it is some aspect of the social environment that is doing it. It could just as well happen randomly, or through their diet or through intrauterine chemical differences during the development of the fetuses that show up later in life. After all, twins cannot occupy exactly the same place in the womb, and would be subject to slightly different intrauterine environmental conditions.

There is the argument that since identical twins are often raised the same way by their parents, it is not surprising that if one twin becomes schizophrenic, the other will also. It is not a genetic matter; it is the same social environment they have been exposed to that is to blame. It is a possibility, but this argument is weakened by certain adoption studies. Normal children of normal parents have, on occasion, been adopted and raised by schizophrenic foster parents. These children are far less likely to develop schizophrenia than the children of schizophrenic parents who have been adopted and raised by normal foster parents. Other studies have shown that the children of schizophrenic parents adopted by normal foster parents are much more likely to be schizophrenic than the children of normal parents adopted by normal foster parents. Therefore, the children of schizophrenic parents are much more likely to be schizophrenic than the children of normal parents regardless of whether these children are raised by schizophrenic or normal parents.

None of those adoption studies was set up as an experiment—it was just data gathering after the fact. A great deal of searching through medical records was necessary to select a sufficient number of cases for further analysis. These studies are not without flaws. It has to be pointed out that the children of schizophrenic parents were seldom adopted immediately after birth, but at some later time. It is possible their natural parents had enough time to influence irreversibly their children's subsequent behavior before they were adopted.

There is no compelling evidence, however, that parents in any way can make their children schizophrenic. There are studies that show the parents of schizophrenics may be different in their behavior than the parents of nonschizophrenics. But any differences can be explained genetically. Any abnormal behavior by these parents may merely mirror the genes shared with their children. If the child behaves abnormally, then it is not surprising that the parents are behaving abnormally to some extent also, since the parents were the source of the genes for the child. While we cannot completely rule out social influences, we cannot completely rule them in either. One test to establish whether there is a truly genetic cause of schizophrenia is unethical and unappealing. Test-tube babies could be made from schizophrenic parents' eggs and sperms and implanted in the uteruses of normal women. After birth they would be raised by their adoptive parents and compared in their incidence of schizophrenia with test-tube babies derived from normal parents grown in the uteruses of schizophrenic women and raised by schizophrenic parents—a rather ugly experiment.

Most schizophrenics do not have a schizophrenic parent, but this does not invalidate the genetic theory. Our genes come, of course, from our parents, but they combine in new ways in developing an organism, or we would all look and behave exactly like our parents. It may be an unusual combination of several genes that produces schizophrenia in offspring, and they all need to be turned on at the same time for the disorder to occur. It may be that a single gene for schizophrenia is carried by one of the parents, but is never expressed or turned on in them as it was for their offspring. We just do not know.

As was illustrated in chapter 2, Figure 8, each gene essentially produces a certain specific kind of protein molecule. These molecules may end up as structural components in our bodies, such as muscles, or may serve as enzymes whose function is to speed up molecular (chemical) reactions in our body. If there is a gene (or genes) for schizophrenia, then the protein molecules produced by it are going to do some damage to our nervous system. In fact, minor nervous-system abnormalities such as coordination and balance difficulties are found in many schizophrenics. They may be due to the medication and nutrition they receive as patients, or these abnormalities may reflect an underlying molecular problem produced by schizophrenia. It is important to remember that even if events in our social environment cause schizophrenia, schizophrenia is still a problem of the molecules because that is what we are made of.

The question we are dealing with in this section is not, as we have seen in the previous chapters, whether this behavior is caused by molecular problems or psychological ones, since all outside influences on us are translated into molecular events. The question is whether psychosocial influences (interactions with other people, places, things, and events), or chemical and physical aspects of our environment (microorganisms, diet, intrauterine influences), or internal molecular events (genes, metabolism), or some combination of all of these cause schizophrenia to develop. We are always influenced by some combination of these as long as we are alive, and it is important to sort them out in order to cure mental illness, as well as to prevent it from occurring.

From a consideration of what we know about schizophrenia, we could conclude that there are genes for it that must be present for the illness to develop. Even though the genes are present, they have to be turned on before schizophrenia develops. If they are turned on by invading microorganisms, or nutritional deficits, or intrauterine influences, or randomly by errors in the molecular machinery, then all the attempts at psychological explanations are pretty much meaningless. We would certainly have to rethink our attitudes about mental illness.

Chemistry of Schizophrenia • Whatever the cause of schizophrenia, the molecular result may be an excess of dopamine molecules in certain nerve cells in the brain. The evidence for this is indirect and not totally certain. Dopamine is a small molecule quite similar in structure to adrenaline (a near relative of which may also be in excess in schizophrenics) and is responsible in some brain cells for conducting the nerve impulse from one cell to another. The chemicals that do this are called neurotransmitters. If too many dopamine molecules are present in certain critical cells, the delicate balance so necessary for normal behavior is disturbed, and disturbed behavior results. If we have a gene for schizophrenia, it would appear to cause the production of too much dopamine in certain brain cells. Dopamine levels are increased by an overdose of amphetamines, which also produce schizophreniclike symptoms in normal individuals. In addition, the molecule chlorpromazine (also called Thorazine), which is used—often quite effectively—to treat schizophrenia, reduces dopamine levels in nerve cells. Autopsies have also revealed that schizophrenics have higher dopamine levels in some parts of their brain than do "normals." These findings support the view that an excess of dopamine molecules causes schizophrenia. Our biochemical makeup comes clearly into view when we consider that a molecule of dopamine is composed of just twenty-two atoms, and may make life pretty miserable for millions of people in the world.

MAJOR DEPRESSION   Feeling depressed for a relatively short time following unpleasant changes in our lives is not at all unusual, and clearly reflects the effects of our environment upon our behavioral chemistry. But when the depression severely interrupts our day-to-day functioning over a long period of time by producing feelings of inadequacy, discouragement, helplessness, and gloominess, then we have a serious illness. Both temporary grief and serious depression, whatever their causes, still reflect underlying molecular changes.

The depression to be discussed here will be severe depression (called major depression by psychiatrists). For the depressed, one could no doubt find events in the past that could have been depressing, such as loss of family, friends, or job, moving, divorce, illness, etc. But these things did not necessarily cause the depression. It is after-the-fact reasoning. Anything can be explained after the fact because there are so many possible explanations that one of them is bound to be appealing. It is like saying we caught a cold because we were very tired, were in a cold draft of air, or got wet feet. Actually we can catch a cold only if someone throws us the cold viruses that cause it. This is easily demonstrated by introducing cold viruses into the nose and throat of volunteers and then watching them sneeze and get a sore throat and runny nose. Try just wet feet and cold drafts of air and nothing of this sort happens. With depression, too, we must be careful about assuming what causes what.

Many who deal with the mentally ill, if they look hard enough, can always find some emotional experience in a person's life to explain the origin of any persistent human behavior, including mental illness. It would not look good to the profession if a clinical psychologist told a patient the problem was molecular. (Nor in all fairness would it look good for a biochemist to claim the problem was your grandmother.) What is lacking is proof that such emotional experiences cause subsequent behaviors. Even if those with depression have been subjected to more genuine depressing experiences, and those with schizophrenia have been subjected to more genuine stress than normal people, this does not establish the cause. As mentioned earlier, this is only one measured difference out of the many possible differences between the normal and the mentally ill. Those depressed and those schizophrenic could each have been exposed to things that normals were not exposed to, such as different microorganisms, different intrauterine environments, or diets that were not adequate for proper brain functioning. Or, as the genetic studies indicate, they may have been different to start with. No one denies that previous emotional disturbances can affect our subsequent behavior, but the claim that they can produce a serious mental illness is in no way proven.

Unlike schizophrenics, those suffering from depression do not come mainly from the lower socioeconomic levels, nor are they found mostly among the divorced or widowed. Thus we can eliminate these conditions as possible causes. Of the more than one and a half million people in the United States being treated for major depression, most are women. Whether this is due to hormonal differences between men and women is not clear, but when something affects one sex more than the other, one becomes suspicious. Between the ages of forty-five and sixty-five we are most likely to suffer depression, but no one can clearly point to earlier psychosocial events as the cause of depression, nor predict who will later suffer from it. Genetic studies have revealed that if one identical twin becomes depressed, the other twin is far more likely to suffer also than if they were fraternal twins. We did see with schizophrenia, though, that these studies may only reflect parents' treating identical twins more similarly than fraternal twins. Adoption studies have indicated, however, that identical twins raised apart by different parents are just as likely to be depressed as identical twins raised together by the same parents. Changing the environment does not reduce the chances of suffering from depression.

Regardless of the cause or causes of depression, the best current guess of what is happening is that there is not enough of the neurotransmitter molecule norepinephrine at the right place in the brain. Norepinephrine is very similar to adrenaline, which—as we know when we "get our adrenaline up"—excites us. If the adrenaline or norepinephrine level gets too low, we slow down and become depressed. If norepinephrine molecules are not present in selected nerve cells in sufficient quantity, nerve signals will not be transmitted from one nerve cell to another at a fast enough rate to maintain a normal level of behavior. Diet may be an important consideration in assuring the availability of the chemical precursors of norepinephrine.

Norepinephrine is synthesized from the amino acid tyrosine. If tyrosine is present in too low an amount in the diet, not enough norepinephrine will be synthesized, and depression may result. If there is a gene for depression, it would act by curtailing the production of norepinephrine in certain cells. The antidepressant drugs (such as imipramine) are thought to increase the availability of norepinephrine at the appropriate nerve cells to speed up nerve impulses. It is like stepping on the gas pedal of a car that is slow and sluggish. While the molecular specifics of major depression are by no means firmly established, they tie in nicely with another mental illness at the other end of depression—mania.

MANIA AND MANIA-DEPRESSION   Of the severely depressed, about twenty percent also show signs of mania, or extreme elation. In mania, the person is overconfident, restless, overactive, and on a "high." Almost everyone who has mania also moves into depression at some time or another. Psychiatrists now call mania-depression a bipolar disorder to indicate its shifting nature. She or he may cycle from one to another every few days or every few months with normal periods in between. If depression is produced by a lack of the norepinephrine molecule, it would be reasonable to guess that mania is produced by an excess of the norepinephrine molecule. Now the gas pedal is pushed to the floor. Lithium carbonate, the drug molecule of choice in treating mania, is thought to decrease norepinephrine levels in certain brain cells. It is not known what causes norepinephrine to ebb and flow within certain critical brain cells. Perhaps it is under the control of an internally generated biological clock; once started, the norepinephrine levels do not seem to be related much to external psychosocial events. That is, the environment has little effect on it.

Some genetic studies suggest that about fifty percent of those suffering from mania-depression may have inherited a gene for it on the X chromosome.* The remaining fifty percent may have a different form of the disorder, possibly not genetic, but molecular nonetheless. Each kind of mental illness has a range of behaviors within

*Humans normally have twenty-three pairs of chromosomes, including an XY pair for males and an XX pair for females. Each chromosome is composed of thousands of different genes.

it that may represent different forms of illness and different causes of it. This may explain why no one drug works on all people, and why some people improve with no help at all. Therefore, classification of schizophrenia and depression into several different types is possible.

ALL TALKING, ALL LISTENING, ALL MOLECULES STILL   The dopamine theory of schizophrenia and the norepinephrine theory of mania-depression as presented here are surely simplified explanations of the underlying molecular events. But, as all the other material in this book suggests, we must give at least equal time to those events before we accept the more traditional psychosocial explanations, which ignore molecular effects.

Ultimately, all our behavior is controlled by molecules, even if the cause of these molecular changes is psychosocial. What we see, what we listen to—what our senses take in—does affect us, but only after being converted into molecular events by our senses. If listening to what is around us hurts us, then talking about it with others could help us. Some forms of mental illness may develop because our thinking has been adversely affected by what our senses take in. Our brain becomes filled with memory molecules that distort our thinking. It is not incompatible with the molecular approach to suggest that talking with a therapist or others can redirect the thinking to cure the mental illness. New memory molecules can replace the old ones. After all, if the psychosocial environment could produce the problem via the senses, an altered psychosocial environment could eliminate the problem via the senses. Words can affect us and our nerve cells (also called neurons). We might change the familiar children's rhyme to read: Sticks and stones may break my bones, but words will hurt my neurons. On the other hand, if the psychosocial environment had nothing to do with causing the illness, then all the talking in the world will not cure the problem. You cannot talk someone out of a disease-produced illness like pneumonia, a vitamin deficiency, or a genetic defect like phenylketonuria. Perhaps there are really just two types of mental illness—those curable by talk and those not.

If one's thinking is fouled up because of faulty learning experiences, then relearning proper responses with the help of others may solve the problem. There are several behaviors resulting from faulty learning experiences, such as fearing situations that offer no threat (phobics), following a strict ritual of meaningless behaviors (obsessive-compulsives), and expecting illnesses that are unlikely to occur (hypochondriacs). Relearning new experiences should help to eliminate these behaviors. However, the faulty thinking resulting from schizophrenia, major depression, and paranoia probably have nothing to do with learning improper responses, and therefore require more than talk. They require direct molecular intervention. Bear in mind, however, that whether your problem is helped by a psychiatrist, a psychologist, a friend, a family member, or by a chemical, they are all redoing your molecules.

GENERALIZED ANXIETY DISORDER A less severe problem than the preceding, but an annoyance nonetheless, is a form of behavior called a generalized anxiety disorder. This disorder is characterized by a variety of symptoms including nervousness, cold and sweaty hands, breathlessness, dizziness, weakness, headache, and an uneasiness about what may happen next. While one could attempt to explain the cause of this anxiety reaction as fear of certain threatening behaviors surfacing from the unconscious, a much more specific explanation is possible. The explanation is molecular. Injecting molecules of lactic acid into the veins of those who have in the past experienced the anxiety disorder, produces anxiety attacks within just a few minutes. The symptoms of these induced attacks cannot be distinguished from those occurring naturally. Lactic acid molecules are present in everyone's body, but when the level gets too high, it is suggested, anxiety symptoms appear. Prolonged, intense exercise produces lactic acid and, in fact, the same symptoms of the anxiety disorder. The difference is that lactic acid increases in the anxiety disorder without exercise.

What gets the levels too high? It is known that an increase of adrenaline in the body leads to an increase of lactic acid production. It is not known what initially increases the adrenaline levels. It may be stress from the psychosocial environment, unconscious brain control, or a faulty gene producing too much adrenaline in certain critical cells.

OPIATES OF THE BRAIN   Only recently has it been discovered that opiatelike substances reside in the brain: They are protein molecules called endorphins (*endogenous morphines*, or the morphine within us). The opiate drugs taken by drug addicts and also prescribed by physicians include opium, morphine, and heroin. They are noted for their painkilling properties as well as for their ability to alter moods. The endorphins, which are part of the brain's natural molecular machinery, appear to function like the opiate drugs, acting as natural painkillers and mood makers. For the heroin addict perhaps there is a little too much pain from life because of insufficient amounts of endorphins in the brain. This can be compensated for by externally supplied painkillers like heroin which deaden the effects of what goes on around the addicts. As far as mental health goes, it has been suggested that the endorphins may play such a major role in regulating moods that disturbances in these molecules could lead to any number of mental illnesses. There is some speculation now that excessive amounts of endorphins may create the moods experienced by schizophrenics. It is too soon to tell, but the endorphins may bring us an important step closer to the causes of molecular madness

Over time, we have seen that more and more thinking disorders are removed from the rather vague classification of mental illness and are being called what they are: genetic, metabolic, nutritional, or infectious disorders of the brain. Their molecular origin is acknowledged. In many cases the role of the psychosocial environment (and the people, places, events, and things in it) in causing mental illness has been lessened or even eliminated altogether, and has been replaced with attention to the role of the chemical and physical environment.

To be sure, mental illness, in all its manifestations, has not been neatly wrapped up in molecular packages. There just are too many research findings that cannot be handled easily by any theory. The same drug may not be effective on everyone suffering from the same mental illness. The molecular theories of mental illness are still tentative, but they offer at least as good an indication of what is happening as do the psychological and sociological theories.

If one really believes that behavior is determined just by molecules, and that the molecules often do things that we cannot control, then an interesting implication arises: Who is responsible for their own behavior and who is not? In the United States and England, for example, those declared insane are not considered to be responsible for their behavior. If they murder someone, they are not legally guilty by reason of insanity. Yet if the insane are not responsible for their behavior, then the sane are not either. Both types are controlled by molecular forces. Molecules in the brain are determining our behavior, and they may go one way or the other—and not at our discretion. Those people who could never murder someone else may have as little control over their behavior as those who insanely murder have over theirs. Either we are all responsible for our behavior or none of us is. Even if an individual is not responsible, societies are. They still decide what should be done, so we are not left in chaos.

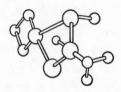

Love and Hate

We love and hate because our molecules tell us to. Both behaviors play important roles in our lives, but let us look at hate first. Hatred expresses itself in many ways in humans, including pushing and shoving, fighting, anger, war, and verbal abuse. It is not clear whether the molecular events leading to all of these acts of aggression are the same or different, so one must be cautious about assuming they have the same biological basis. Those who study aggression must be careful to specify what form of aggression they are dealing with. Aggression will be defined here as purposely doing physical harm to another member of the same species. It excludes, therefore, such behaviors as the hunting and killing of other species for food, aggressive selling tactics, and cursing others. There is no biological distinction between aggression committed illegally by an individual murderer, say, or legally by a soldier acting for his government. Social conditions, not biological ones, determine whether aggression will be committed as a revolutionary, an executioner for the state, or a bomber pilot. Society decides what acts of aggression will be tolerated and which will not, and these decisions often change with the times. If someone is physically harmed on purpose, aggression has occurred. It does not matter to the molecules whether it was done in the line of duty, because we were told to, in self-defense, or for thrills. To be aggressive at any level requires the activation of certain molecules in certain parts of the brain. No activation, no aggression. Some people could never harm someone, others might in self-defense, and still others might enjoy doing so.

RESTRAINTS ON AGGRESSION Aggression as I have defined it does occur among the animals, and has been observed in insects, cats, dogs, rats, monkeys, hyenas, lions, wolves, and apes. Dogs tear each other up on the street much more frequently than wild dogs would ever do in the open. This may be because domestic dogs have a confused sense of territory. Normally there are elaborate behavior rituals many animals go through in the course of fighting that serve to signal the end of the fight—and the prevention of killing. Because members of the same animal species usually avoid killing each other, their fights have been characterized as being more like tournaments. When the going gets too tough, an animal in a fight with one of its own kind may roll over, bow down, or exhibit some other movement to end the aggression. Dogs may signal the end of a fight by lying down, belly up, and exposing their most vulnerable area. In human aggression some such ritual may work, but infrequently. If someone is about to harm you, you could raise your hands to signal surrender and the aggression may stop. But this gesture is less certain to work than a similar one exhibited by animals. Pleading for mercy in front of a gunman, as the newspapers tell us, is not always effective either.

Another way some animals, such as chickens and monkeys, limit their aggression is through a dominance hierarchy. Fighting within the species determines a hierarchy of dominance, placing the animals in rank from most to least dominant. Each one then knows its place with respect to whom it can defeat and who can defeat it: Aggressive acts are decreased. Dominance hierarchies are found in human organizations of all kinds, but with the exception of such groups as street gangs, they are established virtually without any physical fighting at all. For example, the captain is expected to defer to the colonel, the student to the professor, and the foreman to the superintendent.

Human-behavior rituals and dominance hierarchies are less effective than animal ones in limiting aggression, and this fact suggests that other influences also act upon us. In fact, our aggressive responses are modified by learning from the expectations of others just what the proper responses are. Our aggression is also curtailed by laws punishing aggressive behavior. This may be the important difference between animal and human aggression: Our aggression is more subject to modification by the environment. It is very easy to hurt someone with a gun, knife, club, or our bare hands, but we do this infrequently because we have learned not to, and because we may get punished if we do.

FUNCTIONS OF AGGRESSION   Aggression could be useful for an individual in assuring that he or she gets enough of the scarce resources of food, water, and living space, but still not be useful for the species as a whole. If one person stands on tiptoe to view a parade, she can see better; but if everyone does it no one can see any better. Since aggression is widespread among animals, it is necessary to ask whether it has a purpose. Clearly, too much aggression would be harmful to any species, as it would kill itself off. Furthermore, the time spent in aggressive acts could be better spent looking for food, reproducing, and caring for the young. We have seen that behavior rituals and dominance hierarchies function to reduce aggression, presumably for this reason. On the other hand, in animals aggression can lead to the survival of the fittest, where fittest means the best fighter. It does not mean the fittest in all possible ways—the winner may be stupid. If two males are fighting over a female to mate with, the best fighter will be the winner and will pass his genes on to the offspring. There does not necessarily have to be a single gene for aggressiveness that is passed on. There may be several genes that lead to being a good fighter, such as bigger antlers, stronger horns or hoofs, fearlessness, or better eyesight. Similarly, the male that lost the fight—assuming bad luck did not play a part—did not have the proper assortment of genes to win the fight. His relatively inappropriate genes would not be passed on to another generation because he did not have a chance to mate with a female. While such an argument favoring aggression can be made for animals, it is not necessarily the case for humans.

It is not at all necessary now for human males to fight physically over a female for the right to mate with her, although psychological warfare is acceptable and even expected. Choice of mate is based on many attributes besides fighting ability, including looks, intelligence, personality, or availability. Aggression, then, might not be necessary at all now, but it could have been up until about forty thousand years ago, at which time we evolved into our present selves. We may speculate that earlier we were aggressive in the same ways animals were, until the final genetic changes produced our species and eliminated the need for most aggression. After that time, perhaps, language ability, intelligence, or the ability to get along with others became more important. Our aggression may not have been lost, but controls for it may have been added on.

While the kinds of genes we possess have not changed in the last forty thousand years, our way of life certainly has. From that point on we may have needed to cooperate, first to hunt and gather food, and then —about ten thousand years ago—to develop agriculture. Some would even say that agriculture increased our aggressive acts, for now—for the first time—there was territory to defend. Where once there was land for all to walk over and hunt on, now people had worked the land, marked the borders, and were willing to fight to protect their investment.

EVOLUTION OF AGGRESSION   Evolutionary theory tells us that we descended from the animals, and according to one line of reasoning, since animals are naturally aggressive, then we must also be. Actually, one could also make just the opposite argument: Since we evolved from animals we are different from them and are therefore *not* naturally aggressive. The problem, of course, is in determining just what things we have in common with animals that preceded us and just where we differ. We do not look much like them, yet we synthesize protein molecules in the same way, and share common physiological problems, such as getting oxygen molecules to our cells and removing cellular waste products. Whether we are aggressive because we inherited aggressive genes from our predecessors has not been established.

The statistics for crime indicate aggressive acts are present, so whether we are an aggressive species is not an issue—we know we are. In 1976, in the United States, 18,800 murders, 56,700 rapes, and 491,000 assaults were reported (no doubt many more went unreported). Given the population of the United States, about one in four hundred people was physically harmed by an aggressive act by a member of the same species. Many countries have much lower murder rates (Spain, Greece, and Denmark have at least one-tenth the murder rate of the United States) and a few have even higher rates (Puerto Rico and Mexico). These differences are thought to reflect differences in the traditions of these countries and in the way they do things. The created environments may either encourage or discourage violence to one degree or another. The English may expect their males to deal with frustration and hostility with good sportsmanship and grace under pressure. Americans may expect their males to stand up and fight back like their ancestors did who settled this country. What the important factors in the environment are is a matter of dispute: family-rearing practices, poverty, rapidly changing values, television violence, or community morality? There are certainly some genetic differences also among countries that produce differences in such things as the most prevalent blood type and skin color, but it is not known whether other genetic differences exist in these countries that could affect the initiation or control of aggression. We all have perceptions of how we think the people of one country differ in behavior from those of another country: Germans are efficient, Japanese are hardworking, Tahitians are easygoing, etc. Whether these impressions are true is difficult enough to establish, but to try to determine to what extent their behaviors are genetically or environmentally influenced is too formidable a task.

Whether our acts of aggression occur more or less frequently than those of other species of animals, such as monkeys and apes, would also be of interest in telling us whether aggression is on the decrease as we evolve. That is, are we evolving out of it, or are we stuck with it, aggression being as much a part of us as our limbs? Unfortunately, we do not know exactly what mammals we evolved from, so the argument cannot be made that we are aggressive because we evolved from aggressive monkeys or apes, which in turn evolved from the predecessors of rats or mice, or wolves or cats, or whatever. An evolution-ary tree, as in Figure 10, indicates who evolved from whom. If one looks at such a tree for the mammals, it is clear that humans are in quite a distinct category. Humans did not evolve directly from the apes, monkeys, or any other present group of mammals. As Figure 10 shows, humans and apes had a common predecessor, now extinct. Similarly, apes and humans probably did not arise directly from monkeys, but rather shared another common pre-decessor, also now extinct. Consequently, since we do not know if our immediate predecessors were peaceful or ag-gressive, we can make no inference about the evolution of our behavior. It is just as possible that we evolved directly from a most peaceful, cooperative mammal, and that in comparison to the animals around us today, we are not a very aggressive species. We do however become violent about things that do not exist in the animal world, such as money, religion, and politics.

GENES AND AGGRESSION   One thing we do know from evolution is that the most primitive part of our brain (the first part to evolve) is the brain stem. Being the most primitive part, it controls some very basic functions crucial to life: the heartbeat, breathing, and sleep. It has also been found that it initiates aggression. Directly stimulating this part of the brain with electricity will produce aggressive behavior. Over millions of years of evolution, the brain stem has been the most unchanged part of the vertebrate brain. Since the initiation of aggression occurs in a primitive part of our brain, it is a basic function necessary for self-preservation. But most importantly, the aggres-

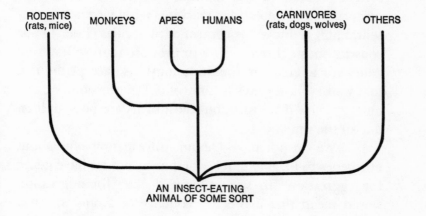

Figure 10: **A POSSIBLE EVOLUTIONARY TREE OF MAMMALS**
Monkeys, apes, and humans are more closely related to each other than to the other mammals. Nevertheless, humans did not evolve directly from monkeys or apes, but through some common ancestor.

sion center in our brain stem does not act by itself (except under laboratory conditions)—it is under the control of a higher and more evolved part of our brain, the limbic system, located in the highest part of our brain, the cerebrum. The molecular machinery for violence is present, but it is under the control of molecules closer to our consciousness. If one wishes to propose that we have the genes for aggression, then one must also accept the fact that we have the genes to control our aggression. We can be aggressive if we wish, but most of us are not—at least not all the time.

We do not have enough information now about our genes to be able to tell whether or not we have genes for aggression. To say we have a gene for aggression would mean that a precise sequence of atoms within a DNA molecule would make us aggressive if the gene were turned on. The gene would make a protein molecule that would in turn activate the aggression area in our brain stem. Such a gene could be turned on (as we saw in the case of some mental illnesses) by an internal molecular event produced at random or by the psychosocial environment after being converted to molecular events by the senses. If there is no gene for aggression, then the environmental input to our senses could directly activate the aggression center of our brain stem and not first have to activate an aggressive gene. Aggression would still be under the control of the limbic system, however.

In any case, learning must still play a role in the expression of aggression. Learning is a higher brain activity and therefore helps play a role in controlling the lower brain activity of aggression. If fighting behavior is rewarded, we are encouraged to fight again. If we are frustrated in doing things, we may learn that being aggressive makes some of us feel better. Since learning has a genetic basis (the production and recall of memory molecules depends partly upon the instructions found in the DNA), the genes determine to some extent how easily we will learn to be aggressive. Furthermore, the higher brain center that controls aggression will also vary in its molecular arrangement from person to person so that the ability to control aggression will also vary among us. Such brain control could influence just how much and what kind of external stimulation is necessary before we become aggressive. Some individuals never become aggressive; others are with only the slightest provocation. Similarly, the genes participating in the development of our body size, senses, and coordination all play a part in determining our propensity to fight and our chances of winning, and thereby fighting again.

It should be apparent that a gene for aggression is not necessary. We can be perfectly aggressive without it. A gene may in fact exist, but we can explain aggression without it. As an analogy, consider language. We learn English or Spanish or whatever—we do not carry a gene for each language. Yet we do have the genes that make language possible. Our lips, tongue, and voice box have to be able to move in certain ways before talking is possible, and our brain has to be capable of symbol (word) manipulation. Other animals do not have these capabilities because the proper genes are lacking. We cannot have genes for everything because there just is not enough room on the DNA. At least we are spared genes for liking fast-food chains, TV situation comedies, and plastic flowers—these things other people have to teach us, and that gives us a chance to avoid them.

One argument against genes being directly responsible for our aggression is that the violent crime rate in the United States and Western Europe is increasing. Yet our genes have not been changing. As we saw, the number of our genes became fixed about forty thousand years ago. The homicide rate (the number of people murdered per one hundred thousand population) in the United States has fluctuated over the years, being twice as high in the 1930s as the 1950s, and generally reaching new highs from 1974 on. Such a change is not really incompatible with having a gene for aggression. We can say not that there are more genes for aggression appearing, but more genes for aggression are being turned on by a changing psychosocial environment (such as more guns being available) or simply by an increase in the number of young people (who commit most crimes). If you will, we have all carried aggressive traits but they are being expressed more frequently because of what is happening around us.

INTERNAL AND EXTERNAL CAUSES OF AGGRESSION   If we learn to be aggressive, then we are learning to respond to certain stimuli in our environment with an aggressive reaction. But it should not be concluded that only external psychosocial stimuli lead to aggression. Unprovoked acts of violence can result from excessive amounts of alcohol, lack of oxygen to the brain, brain tumors, a rabies virus infection, a blow to the head, and

certain kinds of epileptic attacks. Most aggression probably is provoked—at least in the opinion of the aggressor
—by a stimulus from the environment. But as we have
seen over and over, behavior (in this case aggression) can
also be generated independently of surrounding psychosocial events. Furthermore, when certain brain cells are
electrically stimulated by physicians who have inserted fine
wires into them, violent behavior can be produced. When
the stimulation ceases, so does the behavior. Different
people have different thresholds for this stimulation,
suggesting their brain cells would vary in just how much
environmental stimulation they could take until aggression resulted. It is quite possible that these same cells could
be stimulated by molecular events produced by some
disease of the brain. The brain stem itself could be
malfunctioning, or the higher brain center that controls it
could be. A 1979 study of boys at a correctional institution
revealed that virtually all of the most violent boys showed
at least one minor neurological deficit such as a coordination or reflex problem. The deficit was not sufficient to
explain totally their violent behavior, but was symptomatic
of underlying brain damage—damage perhaps to those
brain centers involved in violence and its control. Most of
these violent boys had also been physically abused by their
parents, possibly the cause of their brain dysfunction, or a
contributing factor to it. Since the parents and children
under study both exhibited violence, an inherited tendency for aggression is not out of the question. The boys may
have inherited an inability to handle stressful events and
thus dealt with stress with violence. It is also possible that

the abused boys could have learned to be violent from their parents' example, instead of inheriting anything, and felt it was expected of them to be violent.

Improper brain function could well be the culprit in some forms of violent crime, particularly those committed by mass murderers. These murderers often appear to be tormented in some way by their multiple victims, even though the victims had little or nothing to do with the murderer. The murderers are considered to have terribly faulty perceptions of what is happening around them and by virtually any standard are judged mentally ill. Their brains malfunctioned at random and not because their social environment did it to them.

CRIME AND AGGRESSION   A crime occurs when a law is broken, so the definition of criminality rests with the society that makes the laws. To say that all kinds of crime are committed by born criminals makes no sense, because the genes cannot know ahead of time what behaviors societies will consider to be criminal. Australia, for example, was mostly settled by criminals from Great Britain who were dumped there to rid Britain of some of its undesirables. Yet Australia has a murder rate seven times less than that of the United States. In addition, a crime committed in one country is not punishable in another country. Furthermore, if criminals were merely born that way, then we would expect them to be distributed equally across all segments of society. They are not; in the United States proportionally more criminals are of lower socioeconomic status (a composite measure made up of occupation, income, and education). But a low socioeconomic status (SES) is not sufficient to explain all crime, because in the United States violent crime rates are higher among blacks than Hispanics. Yet both blacks and Hispanics are disproportionally likely to have a lower SES than whites. Furthermore, what may be a crime in one place will not be a crime in another. Casino gambling in Nevada or Atlantic City, New Jersey, is legal, but not in other states. Even if we look just at aggression, sometimes it is a crime, other times not. Bodily assault is legal in the boxing ring, but not in the street unless there is a war going on, when the street is fine. For this reason it is impossible to construct a meaningful biological category describing only aggressive criminals, since some kinds of aggressive people (those who kill in self-defense) are not always categorized by laws as criminals. Likewise, other kinds of people we call aggressive (soldiers who kill in wars) could also be called criminals at another time and place.

If we look at murderers as examples of aggressive people we find that most of the victims were known by the murderers. Furthermore, most killings (when there is no war going on) are the result of a quarrel, and either the killer or the victim most likely has been drinking alcohol. Random killings are the exception rather than the rule, as people most likely kill because they are mad at someone, and they have lost control of their behavior—or maybe they never had control. Have the molecules taken control? In the cases where the killer has had too much alcohol we could reach that conclusion. Alcohol anesthetizes the higher control centers of the brain—those centers that exercise control over aggression. This leaves the brain stem—the initiator of aggression—without proper restraints, and aggressive acts become more probable.

In the United States most murderers are male, black young adults. We must not simply attribute this to the genetics of blacks, because African blacks have much lower murder rates than their descendants, the blacks in the United States. If there were something unique about the blacks' propensity for violence, then wherever there are blacks in the world, violence would be relatively high—but this is not the case. Blacks in Africa commit proportionally fewer murders than whites do in the United States. In fact, even within the United States the murder rate by northern blacks has been less than the murder rate by southern blacks, indicating the environment plays a role.

It is not just the degree of industrialization that leads to violence either. Anthropologists have found murder rates in primitive societies equal to that of industrialized nations. Furthermore, a less industrialized country like Greece has a murder rate twenty times less than that of the USA, while another less industrialized country like Mexico has a murder rate twice that of the USA. Unemployment rates, however, are related to violent crimes for both blacks and whites, though the relationship is greater for blacks. As the unemployment rate for American blacks goes up, so does the rate of violent crime. The expression of violence may be simply a sure way to obtain material goods they do not have and others do. Their frustration and hopelessness in not being treated equal to whites for more than two centuries may, as some researchers have suggested, lead to violence. While everyone is frustrated about something at one time or another, the American blacks with a low SES have many less opportunities to engage in activities that can lessen their frustrations. They cannot go to their suburban country clubs, downtown tennis clubs, summer homes, and leading department stores everywhere to change their environment or shop to forget their troubles. Low SES Hispanics have these frustrations too, but having their own language, a common church, and perhaps a more extended family relationship are thought by some to offer some outlets for frustration and even to restrain violent behavior. Yet if you can see success around you and not share in it, anger can easily develop. We should not be studying blacks in the United States to see why they are violent; we should study whites to see why they make the blacks violent.

Aggressive people show a wide range of motivations for their behavior. For example, the initial motivating molecular events in the brain of the person who kills his or her spouse for an extramarital affair may be quite different from what occurs in the brain of the hired contract killer, or one who kills randomly in a mad shooting spree. They do have in common, though, the same lack of restraint on their aggressive nerve impulses, because most people do not kill. Yet these people share what in most societies would be considered an abnormality. We can look around us and see that aggressive people are abnormal in the sense that they are in the minority and are therefore not "normal." Even in a civil war or revolution, most people are not acting aggressively. What is important to know is whether aggressive people are abnormal only in this statistical sense, or whether they are also abnormal in a molecular sense.

There are any number of ways in which the psychosocial environment is thought to lead to crime. A 1979 study showed that it was possible to predict with some accuracy which adult males would commit crimes against property or against people (aggression) by looking at how they were raised as children. If a parent was aggressive, if there was frequent conflict and disagreement between parents, if the mother had little self-confidence and there was little supervision of the child, then their son would be likely, as an adult, to commit crimes against people. Since these factors do not predict perfectly who will commit crimes and who will not, there is still room for internal biological factors to be involved. Nevertheless, at first glance, these findings suggest a clear environmental cause of criminal behavior. However, if parents were aggressive and argumentative to begin with, the children could have inherited these tendencies. They also could have inherited whatever it is that tends to give people little confidence in themselves (there are plenty of people, who in spite of their success, lack self-confidence). With these inherited characteristics and a lack of parental supervision, a man could drift off into aggressive crimes. A lack of parental supervision and a mother's lack of self-confidence also led to crimes against property.

Additional factors contributing to this kind of crime by men were a lack of a mother's affection toward the son and a father's deviance (alcoholism or a criminal conviction). As you will see later in this chapter, affection or love has a biological basis so the son could have inherited a general lack of love for others, and hence have no reason to refrain from taking advantage of others. If the son's father is a criminal (as the next section will show) the son may have inherited some general tendency to engage in antisocial behaviors. What I am saying then is that some child-rearing practices that appear to influence subsequent behavior can be explained away by what the child has inherited from his parents.

For a certain kind of person, aggression may be the only way to deal with a particularly troublesome situation—for example, assaulting someone to obtain money or power over others. Learning may play a large role also. Aggressive criminals may not have learned or accepted the relatively nonviolent standards or values of the larger society in which they live. Or, contact with other aggressive people in an environment where aggressive behavior is rewarded may lead to aggression. They may in fact feel in this case that their society is a violent one. Changing values and the social disorganization of a person's life brought on by such things as crowding, unemployment, a broken home, or parental neglect have also been suggested as leading to aggression. Such disorganization is thought to lead to frustration, which is relieved by aggression.

While these are all reasonable explanations of aggression, it is very difficult to prove them. As we saw with mental illness, the only way to prove the relevance of environmental factors is to subject children and adults to these conditions and observe whether they become more aggressive than others not subjected. This of course is not possible or desirable. We know that only a small percentage of people exposed to these environmental conditions react aggressively, so something is unique about the molecular structure of their brain that leads them and not others to aggression. By no means are most poor people at the bottom of society aggressive. Aggressive people may have a brain that does not learn how to inhibit aggressiveness or a brain that initiates aggression too easily. It has been suggested that the habitual criminal's brain has a distorted time sense in that he or she thinks mostly about the present and does not think about being apprehended in the future. If he is poor, he may think he has no future anyhow. Furthermore, the molecular responses that produce fear in others may be working less well in the habitual criminal. With much less fear of getting caught, more chances are taken and more attention can be focused on the crimes themselves.

GENES AND CRIME   Where might these molecular abnormalities come from? Some studies done in Denmark on crime rates in adopted children show just how both inheritance and the environment interact to produce the problem. The crimes studied are not all crimes of aggression, so we must remember some of the problems in studying crime. As Table 1 indicates, children of noncriminal fathers who are adopted by stepfathers—some of whom are criminals and the rest not—show the same crime rate when they grow up. If the predisposition (inheritance in a general sense) is not there, then it makes no difference whether the children were raised in a criminal or noncriminal environment. It is not known

Table 1: CRIME, HEREDITY, AND ENVIRONMENT

Children of Noncriminal Fathers	adopted by	Criminal Stepfathers	produce	Average Crime Rate
Children of Noncriminal Fathers	adopted by	Noncriminal Stepfathers	produce	Average Crime Rate
Children of Criminal Fathers	adopted by	Noncriminal Stepfathers	produce	Higher Crime Rate
Children of Criminal Fathers	adopted by	Criminal Stepfathers	produce	Highest Crime Rate

(Derived from data from "Criminality in adoptees and their adoptive and biological parents: a pilot study," in *Biosocial Bases of Criminal Behavior* edited by S.A. Mednick and K.O. Christiansen, Gardner Press, New York, 1977)

what this predisposition to crime might be, but it was suggested above that learning or perceptual difficulties may be a part of it. However, if the inheritance was there and children of criminal fathers were adopted and raised by noncriminal stepfathers, a higher crime rate occurs with these children later. Given the same inheritance from a criminal father, but now adoption by a criminal stepfather, the crime rate of the children is at its highest. The unfavorable environment that stepfathers bring to the children in the form of encouragement and support, plus the inheritance of the children, produce the highest crime rate.

There is not a gene for crime; this has already been ruled out. What is thought to be inherited is a combination of genes that leads to antisocial behavior, but what the actual combination might be is not known. What is antisocial behavior in one circumstance may be acceptable in another. Pushing people around at a party is antisocial behavior, but doing it on a wrestling mat is not. Therefore, something like the desire to engage in physical activity regardless of the situation may be genetically transmitted. Maybe the children inherited a somewhat faulty memory that prevents them from learning what not to do. The criminal may inherit a tendency to be impulsive, to act before the consequences are well thought out.

Perhaps, as we saw, the criminal's time sense is distorted, so that attention is paid only to present rewards and not to punishment in the future. Our sense of time is brain based (see chapter 3), depends upon molecular events, and potentially is inheritable. If we couple these behavioral tendencies with the appropriate environment, criminality in the form of antisocial behavior may result. The crimes these factors might apply to include aggressive crimes like assault, rape, murder, and other ones like kidnapping for ransom and armed robbery. It does not apply to crimes like breaking the law by parking illegally, letting your dog run loose off the leash, crossing against a red light, or betting illegally. People who commit other crimes like fraud, embezzlement, forgery, and shoplifting may fall somewhere in between having some inheritable behavior component and having none.

The kind of adoption study in Table 1 is done on a small scale after the fact, because both criminal and adoption records must be searched to pull out the records of people appropriate for the study. The children are not purposely given up for adoption to criminal stepparents. The adoptions were coincidental and were discovered after the fact in public records. The studies followed. The criminal stepfathers had to be matched as closely as possible with the noncriminal stepfathers in terms of their age, the age of the child at adoption, where they live, etc. This eliminates other explanations of the results, such as saying criminal stepfathers adopted their children earlier than noncriminal stepfathers, and thereby had more influence in leading them to crime. These studies are not without fault, and there are just too few of them to be conclusive—but they are suggestive. They suggest the internal molecular state of a person is just as important as the social processes going on around him or her.

It is not an easy matter to relate genes to crime, as experience with the statistically abnormal XYY males has indicated. A human male normally has two sex chromosomes (genes make up chromosomes) designated as XY (a female also has two, designated as XX). The X chromosome always comes from the mother's egg and the Y chromosome can only come from the father's sperm, if a male (XY) child is conceived. If a female child (XX) is conceived, one X comes from the mother's egg and the other X comes from the father's sperm. Eggs always contribute an X chromosome, but sperm may contribute an X or Y. Clearly, the Y sex chromosome determines maleness. In about one in two thousand male births, an XYY child will appear (XXY males and XXX females also infrequently appear) as a result of a developmental abnormality.

In 1965 it was reported for the first time that in a

hospital for the criminally insane there was a disproportionate number of XYY males than would be expected on the basis of how many there were in the general population. One in twenty-eight of the patients was an XYY, yet the general population outside of jail had only about one in two thousand XYY's. Subsequent studies throughout the world in mental institutions, prisons, jails, and detention centers confirmed the finding: XYY males were likely to be criminals. Careful examination of arrest records eventually revealed that their crimes were very frequently against property and not against people. They were not aggressive as we defined it, as they hurt no one; so being an XYY has nothing to do with having genes for aggression. As it turns out, it may have nothing to do with criminality either. The XYY male typically has a lower IQ than an XY male, and because of this may be less clever in avoiding the police and arrest. There is also some evidence that XYY's are impulsive and do not think through their actions. They have clues and more XYY's arrested. As I have said, there cannot be a genetic basis for criminality per se, only for other behaviors that can lead to antisocial acts if the environment is just right. The hints are here, though, that some criminals—aggressive or not—are physiologically different, whether it be their intelligence, memory, personality, or other brain functions, and this some think makes them more likely to behave in ways that most countries would call criminal.

HORMONES AND AGGRESSION Male mammals are generally more aggressive than females. We can manipulate sex-hormone levels in males and females and demonstrate that male aggressiveness is not just the result of learning. Castrating male animals reduces male testosterone levels and significantly reduces aggression. Injecting these same hormone molecules back into the castrates restores their aggressive behavior. Injecting testosterone into adult noncastrated males also causes aggression. Frequent injections of testosterone hormone molecules into adult female animals will increase their aggressiveness to equal that of males. If male sex hormones increase aggressiveness, would female sex hormones (estrogens) decrease it? In animals, giving estrogens to adult males does not reduce their aggressiveness, perhaps because the male sex hormones have been asserting their effects for so long. But if estrogen is given to males soon after birth and subsequently, the males become less aggressive, for now there has been sufficient time for the female sex hormones to neutralize part of the male sex-hormone influence during development.

Some of the hormones of the adrenal glands, located over each kidney, also play a role in aggression. These hormones are known as the adrenal steroids and include the well-known cortisone molecule, which is used as an anti-inflammation drug. Removing the adrenal glands from male animals decreases aggressiveness, but injecting the animals with adrenal steroid molecules increases it again. Just injecting these hormones into normal adult animals will increase aggressiveness. Steroid levels in the blood also increase during aggressive acts. When an animal stops being aggressive because it has been defeated in a fight, some other hormone levels change also. After all, if some molecules cause aggression, others could well stop it. After a male mouse has lost a fight with another male, the injection of a brain hormone (vasopressin) causes the defeated mouse to be submissive in other fighting encounters for up to seven days. Without the hormone treatment, mice are back fighting again within two days. The aggression and submission produced by the injected hormones are not strange forms of behavior, but the same kinds of behavior that normally occur.

Whether these hormone effects upon animal aggression are identical with what occurs in humans is not known, but in humans they would surely be not quite so simple. No one needs to be reminded that we are different from animals in some ways, but remarkably similar in other ways. When we develop laws to ban cancer-causing agents, we accept that what causes cancer in animals can cause cancer in us. It is a no greater act of faith to expect that chemical studies of aggression in animals will reveal facts not too different from those we would find in humans.

WOMEN AND AGGRESSION   Studies on human females and aggression appear to corroborate the animal studies: Males are more aggressive than females. The rate of violent crimes committed by women in the United States has not increased significantly from 1960 to 1977. Furthermore, for most countries in the world where there is data, we can say that the homicide rate for females is virtually always lower than that for men. This all leads to the conclusion that women are physiologically different than men when it comes to aggression. Hormones are the reason, if we can infer from animal studies.

We must say that the human female brain again differs from that of the male (we saw another difference in chapter 3). The difference is in the brain structures and molecules that initiate and control aggression. In contrast to violent crime, the female nonviolent crime rate in the United States is increasing, suggesting that more opportunities for crime are available. As women enter new jobs they will now have a chance to embezzle funds from a corporation or sell worthless real estate just like men do. The crime increase for women is not due to just these activities it is thought; it probably owes more to increased welfare fraud, shoplifting, and passing bad checks and credit cards. As women become more liberated in their thinking they may well say to themselves, "If men can commit crimes, why can't women do it also?" Yet women stop short of increasing their violent crimes because their molecules stop them.

NEUROTRANSMITTERS AND AGGRESSION We saw in the previous chapter that the molecules (the neurotransmitters) that play a role in transmitting nerve impulses between nerve cells have important effects upon our mental health. It is not surprising then that neurotransmitters are important in another aspect of our mental health—namely, aggression. The neurotransmitter molecule acetylcholine has been injected directly into selected areas of animal brains and has caused aggressive behavior. Rats that normally would not kill a mouse brought into their cage would now kill after injections of this neurotransmitter. Conversely, if the acetylcholine that normally is in the brain is chemically blocked in the brain of rats that normally kill mice, then these rats will not kill mice. Attacking a member of another species is not strictly within our definition of aggression, which was restricted to interactions within a single species. In fact, the neurotransmitter-induced aggression has all the actions of predator-prey attack, for the chemically stimulated rats kill the mice in a very sterotyped way—exactly as they would if they were out of the laboratory setting. The injected neurotransmitter must be initiating nerve impulses whose generation has been programmed into the brain to lead to attack behavior.

Similarly, aggression—as we have defined it—may also depend upon a neurotransmitter being released at a specific brain site. Its release would be caused by the psychosocial environment or by brain events independent of the environment. Let us imagine that a threatening situation develops. We see what is happening (someone is coming at you with fists clenched!) and nerve impulses from your eyes are sent to the brain. Here, what these nerve impulses represent is compared with what is stored in memory from past experience as being threatening. If they match, an aggressive response will be initiated, so another kind of nerve impulse is transmitted by a neurotransmitter molecule to the aggressive center of the brain. You now clench your fists and begin to hit.

LOVE   Just as molecules cause aggression, so too do they produce feelings of love. But it is rather too bad that we know a lot more about the biology of aggression than we know about the biology of love. While we can see examples of love all around us, it is not obvious just what to look for that would distinguish at the molecular level when we love someone from when we do not. Love is not simply the biological opposite of hate, nor are there love molecules any more than there are hate molecules. Rather, several different kinds of molecules acting on certain specific brain cells probably produce these feelings, as was the case with aggression.

Lovesickness, the feelings that come over us when we are away from someone with whom we are madly in love, is an example of the changes in our body that accompany love. The loss of appetite, sleeplessness, light-headedness, and single-minded concentration toward the loved one are all real effects caused by physiological changes, molecular in nature. If we love someone we usually express it with actions: kissing, hugging, caressing, and doing nice things. We also do these things for those we like a lot, although with less intensity. Therefore there is not always a clear distinction in our actions between liking and loving, even though we know there is a real difference in our feelings. Aggression, by contrast, was easy to distinguish as a unique behavior because it involved harming others, period. In looking at the biology of love, we can deal with two well-studied aspects of it: parental behavior and altruism.

PARENTING   In most mammal species, the females do most of the parental care of the young. Rather than merely choosing to do it, they may be moved to do it by their genes and the molecules the genes control. The female mammal may spend more time parenting than the male because by the time her infant is born, she has already invested the entire gestation time in her offspring. By contrast, the male has only spent a few minutes of time in creating the offspring, and then he is off. Nursing her infant, the female adds more time to her investment. To protect her high-cost investment, the female may not wish to risk having the male—who considers it a low-cost, low-yield investment—do the parenting. Lest we drift off into a discussion of personal finance, we must add that the male cannot be sure he is the father in the certain way the female knows she is the mother. He presumably should not spend time caring for children not his own.

The point of caring for children after all is to insure that one's genes are perpetuated. Animals, humans included, do not have offspring just to have someone nice around the house. Anyway, children are not all that nice. They do not do what they are told, they make unpleasant noises, they are messy, and they take time and effort. The requirement to perpetuate oneself is present in all forms of life, including bacteria and viruses. Whenever the conditions are right (whether it be sexual desire in humans, estrus—heat—in animals, the chemical environment for bacteria and viruses, or the amount of light for plants), all living things will attempt to reproduce. It is not simply that we choose to reproduce; we are compelled to by our molecules to have the species continue. Placing a birth-control barrier between male and female does not diminish this basic compulsion to engage in reproduction, since sex is a reproductive act. Reproductive acts give the most pleasurable physical feelings possible. The pleasure is the motivating factor or compulsion to perform reproductive acts. In a way, all love can be considered sexual if we look at love as one of those behaviors that also helps perpetuate the species as does sex. If we love friends, we do not harm them and injure our species. If we love our children, we help them safely reach reproductive age. If we love our relatives, we help those with whom we share common genes. The end (survival) justifies the genes (sexual behavior).

Let us not assume that animals other than humans consider the information available and then make a decision about what to do for parental care. The decision has been built into their molecules. As with any type of behavior, there is a genetic basis for the pattern of parental care. The variability among species is enormous, however. Using just the insects as an example, both parents in one stingless bee species ignore their young. In some beetle species, both parents care for the young. In some crickets, it is the female who handles the parental care; in some bugs (contrary to popular usage this is a distinct insect category) it is the male.

It would be interesting to know to what extent parental-care behaviors are built into the human female. Mothers in the United States do more of the child care than the fathers, but since World War II more and more mothers relinquish this care to relatives and day-care centers. So if there is any molecule that may bind mothers to care directly for their children, it can easily be escaped from by human females. But mothers, like fathers, still feel responsible for providing care for their young. This is an expression of love, even if someone else does some of the child care for them. Not all parents care for their young; we still have examples of child abuse and infanticide. By and large these behaviors suggest something is wrong with the molecules controlling our love responses. However, among those people of the world near starvation, killing infants does have survival value for older children in the family. Reducing the demands on a limited food supply protects the investment in time and effort the parents have made in the older children who are closer to the reproductive age. Their new crop of children can then help them out. Nevertheless, our species has survived because enough children have been cared for long enough for them to be parents themselves, and so repeat the cycle. The care of children (either by parents or others) is so important it cannot be left to our cultures to teach us to want to care for them. Cultures certainly tell how to care for children, but the desire to care for them must come from our genes. We cannot as a species take a chance that we will not want to care for our offspring.

Molecules are made and released from our brain under the control of the genes that make us want to take care of our young. What these molecules are for humans we do not know. We do know something about them in animals. Virgin male and virgin female rats will eventually show maternal behaviors when presented with nonrelated newborn rats, so there is some basic compulsion to care for the young. This behavior can be markedly speeded up by injecting the females and males with a variety of sex-hormone molecules. Virgin female rats can also be induced to produce maternal behaviors if they are given a transfusion with the blood from lactating female rats. Nursing mice will make a greater effort than when not nursing to reach their young if separated from them.

Clearly something is going on inside animals that directs them to care for their young. One may get the impression that all there is to life is to perpetuate life.

It has been observed that if the mother-infant relationship in apes and humans is broken at some critical time in the infant's first year, the infant is likely to show behavioral problems later in life. The child may fail to trust others and may avoid close interpersonal contacts. On the other hand, if the infant has had a close relationship with its father, siblings, or other relatives, the interruption of the mother-infant relationship has less of an effect. In any case it seems to be required by its molecules that an infant attach itself to someone: Love has survival value. From an evolutionary perspective, those parents without the genes for love would have fewer surviving children, since the offspring would not be sufficiently cared for. Over time the loveless would decrease. Those with these "love genes" would have more surviving children to pass the genes on to subsequent generations, and so perpetuate this aspect of love.

ALTRUISM   Another expression of love is concern for others, and when it is such that an individual helps another at risk to itself, it is called altruism. If a prairie dog sees a coyote approaching its colony, it calls out an alarm to warn the others, even though the noise makes its location known to the coyote. An adult who rushes into a burning building to save others is acting altruistically. Why does this happen? Do we learn to be nice, to love others to this extent? Probably not, for this behavior too is in our genes. In terms of evolution, it is in our own best interest to assure the survival of those closest to us genetically, so we should be most altruistic toward our closest relatives, with whom we share the most genes. Altruistic behavior would be beneficial if one risked his or her life to save several near relatives. Risking one's life for a stranger offers no such advantage, particularly if the stranger is unlikely to be in a position to help you later. However, trading a near relative's life for another's accomplishes nothing in the preservation of the species unless those who are past reproductive age save those capable of reproduction. In other words, there is benefit if one saves many near relatives or if the old save related young. We can still be altruistic toward strangers when we risk our life for theirs because the genes directing our behavior cannot distinguish between relatives and strangers. In our evolution, we may have interacted much more with relatives than with strangers, and it was a problem of either helping relatives or not. Those who did help those with similar genes helped the survival of the species.

One can get the impression that all the forms of love we express have a genetic basis, because love is caring for others, and this is beneficial to the preservation of the species. We can learn to love others, and we do, but the molecular machinery that makes love a possibility must be there first. Parents may teach such things as decency, generosity, respect, and kindness to their children not so much to have them fit better into society as to help themselves (the parents) survive a little bit better. It is said the parents gain by this behavior maybe more than their children. Over the course of evolution, those who did not love and care for their offspring had their offspring die.

Those with the genes for love had surviving offspring who would then pass on these genes to their young.

SOCIOBIOLOGY   Love and aggression, in all their manifestations, are behaviors directed at someone else, and in a sense are not observable when someone else is not around. These are sociological behaviors because they involve the two or more people interacting. In contrast, most of the other behaviors discussed in this book require no one else to set off the behavior. These are psychological behaviors because they pertain to an individual. If we look at the biological origins of psychology, we have a field of study called psychobiology; and if we look at the biological origins of sociology we have sociobiology. Sociobiologists study human societies and psychobiologists study individuals—from a biological perspective.

Sociobiologists claim that there is a significant biological basis for our social behaviors, like love and aggression. The counterclaim is that social behaviors are learned from the culture. This, of course, is the same old debate of whether our genes or our environment contribute the most to shaping our behavior. It should be clear from discussion in this book that both factors can contribute to behavior, but most often one contributes more than the other. Nevertheless, this debate has importance because of its implications for public policy making. If one believes the sociobiologists, their opponents argue, then one must accept our behaviors as they are and not expect to change them by changing society. Therefore, prison rehabilitation programs for aggressive criminals, laws to punish aggression, more police on the streets, monetary aid to cities to eliminate unemployment and frustration, and training programs to prevent child abuse would have little effect upon reducing aggression. In political terms, putting government funds into special projects would not improve our behavior very much. This is not good news to the molecules of those who have faith in using government programs to improve society.

Even if the sociobiologists are right, it does not mean we have to accept the status quo. It just means we have to deal with our problems in other ways, using biological rather than social tools. We do not accept all of what our biology or genes have given us anyway. We replace kidneys, hearts, teeth, and eye lenses. We throw out tonsils, appendixes, cancerous breasts, and gallstones. We inject allergin molecules into ourselves to control allergies and insulin molecules to control diabetes. Now you say this is not changing behavior, only our bodily structures to save or improve our life. But people's behavior does change after these procedures, particularly if they would have been dead without a new heart or kidney or insulin treatment! The pain from a toothache is going to affect our behavior; so is not being able to see because of cloudy eye lenses (cataracts). The point of all the medical procedures is to improve our behavior by giving us the chance to do some things with a healthy body.

These medical procedures, which are so much a part of our life, are individually decided upon and not imposed upon someone by someone else, like the government. Yet governments at all levels are always trying to change our behavior with laws and punishments, tax incentives, and government-funded programs. Even such simple, everyday things as traffic stop signs, fences, church sermons, and magazine advertisements are there to control or influence our behavior. Most people pretty much accept these attempted influences and controls; in fact they probably keep us all civilized by giving order to society. But when these controls on our behavior fail to work, when the rate of violent crimes goes up, when wars continue to be fought, when basic human rights are denied, and when people care less and less about each other, one begins to wonder if the social tools are working. Of course the social reformers could say that we still do not have the right social programs, or that we have not spent enough money on the ones we do have. The sociobiologists could say it is now the time to consider using biological tools to directly change our behavior. In the future, it will be interesting to see which way unwanted social behaviors are going to be changed.

We do not love just to be nice to others, and we do not become aggressive just to be mean. The vampire bat and the leech suck our blood not to harm us, but in order to survive (the English playwright George Bernard Shaw said this was also true of literary critics). We do these things because they have been advantageous to our survival and are part of our molecular structure. If we love others, we help our species survive, and if we are aggressive we help ourselves survive. There is not a gene for love or one for aggression or criminality any more than there is a gene for flying. Rather there are many genes whose molecular products can lead to these behaviors. We have the molecular machinery to love or to harm, but we can learn to go in one direction or another if our brain is functioning properly. If not, if there are genetic defects in our ability to learn to control love and hate, if microorganisms have invaded the brain, if the proper nutrients do not reach it, or if the molecular integrity of the brain is otherwise violated, then we can expect an absence of love or an excess of aggression.

6

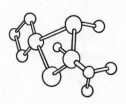

Molecular Self-Improvement

Why do some of us get too fat, drink too much, get unhappy too often, not follow the sexual life-style expected of us, get ground down by stress, or have generally unattractive personality traits? Did our parents do something wrong in raising us, did we come under the bad influences of others, or did events around us misshape us? To be sure, not every overweight, drunken, homosexual, burdened, or unpleasant person is unhappy, nor are those who have everything going for them necessarily happy. To what extent might we have a molecular excuse for aspects of ourselves that we do not like? Just how much can we expect to change ourselves by our good intentions? It may be more difficult than we imagine because to change ourselves we have to change our molecules. Molecules seldom respond to good intentions. Your molecules are your own worst enemy; on the other hand they can be your best friend.

OVEREATING   Weighing more than you should for your sex, height, and age would qualify you as overweight. Weigh twenty-five percent more than you should and you are obese. In any case, if you do not eat much you do not get fat. To do so would violate the first law of thermodynamics: You cannot get something (fat) for nothing (not eating). A word to the size is sufficient. People in World War II concentration camps in Germany and Japan did not get fat. People in famine areas do not get fat.

It is known that amphetamine drugs reduce food intake, consequently they are used as diet pills. Amphetamine molecules, besides doing other things, apparently bind to nerve cells in the appetite centers of the brain and prevent nerve impulses from being generated that would signal the feeling of hunger to us. If the appetite centers are blocked, we will not feel hungry. Phenylpropanolamine is a molecule similar in structure to the amphetamines, and it too has an appetite-suppressor effect. Phenylpropanolamine also acts as a decongestant and is found in a variety of nonprescription cold and allergy remedies.

Many drugs have multiple effects. One is reminded of the story of the scientist who invented a drug that not only cured hemorrhoids, but also could be used as a food seasoner. He put some on his spaghetti dinner once and it tasted good; only trouble was, it shrank his meatballs. Other kinds of molecules within our body, the endorphins (discussed in another context in chapter 4), may serve to increase eating. Naturally occurring endorphin molecules in the brain can be released into the bloodstream, targeted for the stomach. Here the endorphins may block the nerve impulses from the stomach that tell the brain the stomach is full, and we continue to eat. Norepinephrine applied to the brain will cause hunger in "full" animals.

There are two major factors in overeating: food intake and food metabolism. They are interrelated, since some people can eat a great deal and never gain much weight, while others can eat less and gain. As far as food intake goes, there is some suspicion that those who grossly overeat (and there are seven million of us in the United States) are not receiving the proper nervous-system signals from their digestive systems to indicate that enough food has been taken in. Usually we know when we are full because the bulk in our stomach stimulates nerves to send impulses to our brain. Those who overeat may get these signals a little late, after too much food has been eaten, and we all know what a little extra food every meal adds up to—too much. The brain also receives chemical signals from the stomach via the bloodstream. A protein molecule called cholecystokinin may be one of the signals that indicates when we have eaten enough. Obese mice have three times less of this molecule in their brains than nonobese mice. Furthermore, injecting this molecule into sheep and mice causes them to reduce their food intake. Another kind of naturally occurring protein molecule, calcitonin, will also inhibit eating when injected into rats and monkeys. In addition, it has been shown that when food is introduced directly into the human stomach via a surgically implanted tube, the patient still feels hungry. The same amount of food taken by mouth would make her feel full. The conclusion is that if the throat is not properly stimulated with food, hunger can result. For some, the interaction of food molecules with nerve cells in the stomach or throat may not be sufficient to generate nerve impulses or release cholecystokinin or calcitonin to lead to stopping food intake. The absence of the proper molecular signals leads to overeating.

The other major factor in overeating is the body's metabolism, the assembly and disassembly of molecules for use in the body. Our metabolism is influenced both by internal chemical events and by demands put upon the body. Exercise, an example of the latter influence, speeds up our metabolism. In molecular terms, exercise speeds up the demand for energy for muscle use, and metabolism supplies this energy. The internal events affecting metabolism are those created by enzyme molecules, which control what happens to all the kinds of food in our body. Figure 11 illustrates the essentials of the metabolism of overeating.

The food we eat is composed mostly of water, protein, fat, and carbohydrate molecules (vitamins and minerals are a very small portion of the total). Proteins, fats, and carbohydrates represent three distinct classes of molecules, which can be characterized by certain distinct properties. Proteins are very large molecules compared to the other two. Of the remaining two, carbohydrates (sugars) dissolve in water, while fats do not. This is why, for example, the greasy fats we get on our hands during cooking do not just wash off in water. Enzymes in the mouth and stomach attack the food molecules and break them down into smaller and smaller molecules having a different chemical structure. In so doing, the energy that held these large molecules together is liberated, and is utilized by our cells to move muscles, to produce nerve impulses, and to keep the cells alive. Eventually all the available energy is extracted by the cells. One substance that is formed as a waste product with no available energy left in it is carbon dioxide, which eventually reaches the lungs via the bloodstream and is exhaled. In addition, water is excreted as urine and as part of the feces. Other molecular waste products end up in the feces or urine also.

The energy-extraction process that is part of our metabolism is done in many steps in our body. Figure 11 simplifies the molecular breakdown of proteins and fats but shows that they can eventually enter the same chemical pathway that carbohydrates follow. In molecular terms, what this means is that the chemical structures of proteins and fats are rearranged by enzymes and simplified by removing atoms of one kind and another until they have the same chemical structure as the carbohydrates do. In other words, proteins and fats in our foods are transformed into carbohydrates, and their energy is extracted. Proteins may also be broken down into their component parts, the amino acids, to be rebuilt later into new kinds of proteins. Fats may also be rearranged in chemical structure to use in the membranes of cells. Metabolism allows an organism to convert types of molecules it does not need (but has available because it has eaten them) into those it does need. A horse, after all, is made of plants.

Normally, fats in the diet either get deposited in the tissues as fat or have their energy extracted from them, thereby converting them into carbohydrates and eventually eliminating them from the body. If too much fat stays in your body, then you are fat. When there is an

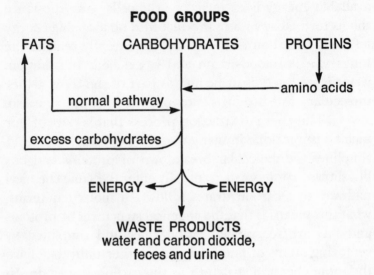

Figure 11: DIGESTION OF FOOD AND
FAT PRODUCTION
*Energy can be extracted from all the food groups until nothing
is left except waste products, which are excreted from the body.
Carbohydrates in excess of what the body needs at any given
time can be converted to fats and stored.*

excess of carbohydrates in the diet, some of the carbohydrates are converted into fats for storage (see Figure 11), and the rest end up with their energy extracted for cellular use. The "wisdom of the body" is not to waste food taken in, but rather to store it for future use—fat is the storage medium. Exercise demands more energy from the body, and during exercise the excess fat follows the normal pathway of energy extraction to supplement what energy can be extracted from the carbohydrates in the body. Figure 11 demonstrates simply why eating excess carbohydrates and not exercising much can lead to obesity. There are no fat marathon runners, even though they may load up on carbohydrates before running.

Enzymes control each step in the digestion of food; it may be that for those tending to gain weight, the enzymes converting carbohydrates to fats may be a little too quick to act. Likewise, for those without weight problems, these converting enzymes may be a little slow to function, so little fat is laid down. Another way to say this is that those who are thin use up their carbohydrates and fats more readily or pass them out as waste faster than do those who are fat. Furthermore, the obese may have faulty enzymes that do not allow their fats in storage to be metabolized at a fast enough rate to offset the adding on of new fat. Those that just tend to put on a few extra pounds of weight also have these enzymatic problems, but to a lesser extent. For females, there is an additional consideration. They have almost twice as much body fat as males do. As simple and pleasurable observation reveals, most of the excess fat is stored in the thighs, breasts, and buttocks. This fat gives them energy reserves for childbearing.

Whenever there is a metabolic reason for a behavior, enzymes are always involved because they control the speed of metabolism in the body. Enzymes are always protein molecules, and proteins are made under the direction of the genes (DNA). If DNA is involved, then we have a genetic basis for the behavior. Therefore, differences in DNA in different people lead to the production of different metabolic enzymes, which lead to differences in body weight. The obese, as compared to the merely overweight, either have more of these metabolic problems or have one of them in greater severity. Since obese strains of mice can be bred in the laboratory, we know DNA and the metabolic pathways it controls are involved in overeating. It is said that fat people tend to run in families, but so do dirty dishes, so a fat family is not sufficient evidence in itself for an inherited predisposition, although it is consistent with one. The children may have learned to eat like the parents. Fat people, it is observed, also have fat pets (we can safely rule out inheritance here), perhaps because in having more food around, the people have more scraps to give away. Alternatively, fat people may have a different standard of body weight and not think of themselves or their pets as fat (others are too thin). They may regard a heavier body weight as more attractive and healthy. If so, then the fat are fat because they choose to be, not because they are compelled to be fat by their metabolism. Whatever genetic components there may be to overeating, we can still overcome them by eating less, by learning to eat less fattening foods, and by exercising. The increase in obesity in the last few decades in the United States is due to people ignoring these three factors.

There is no accepted psychological profile of fat people that would indicate what personality traits lead to overeating. If studies with rats are any guide, it is not simply learning to like fattening foods like sugar as a child that does us in as adults. Early in life rats can eat a large amount of sugar (sucrose) in their diets, but as they pass puberty they eat no more sugar than rats given little or no sugar when young. At least in rats, eating a lot of sugar when young will not predispose them to eating a lot of sugar when reaching adulthood. The fat do not seem to eat more because of stress than do the thin: they are not eating more to compensate for any problems they might have. We are left with no demonstrable psychosocial cause of excessive overeating. It does not mean there is not one, but it makes the molecular explanations that much more attractive. If you have trouble losing weight, the molecular gods are against you.

There seems to be no end to the number of diet plans that are published, and given the number of foods and food combinations that are possible, there will not be an end to them. But for any diet to work, it must follow the logic of Figure 11. This is how our metabolism works, and to deny it in our eating habits is going to cause us trouble with our weight. The only way to lose weight is to eat less food totally, eat less fattening foods, or exercise. Where there is a will, there is less to weigh. The most popular diet plans are those that make this all as painless as possible. Eventually we may even be able to control our weight by eating along with our food the enzymes that would convert unneeded food into waste products, and prevent it from being stored as fat. Sprinkle on some "Dietzyme" or

"Digesto" and eat all you want! The food will taste good but it will move out quickly.

ANOREXIA NERVOSA   An eating disorder just the opposite of overeating is anorexia nervosa, a form of self-induced starvation. It occurs most frequently in girls aged twelve to sixteen, with a frequency of occurrence possibly as high as one in two hundred girls of this age in Western countries. This disorder is characterized by a purposeful sustained weight loss greater than twenty-five percent of the normal body weight, and is accompanied by a fear of being fat (even after the weight loss). In females, menstruation also stops.

Anorexia is the diagnosis when there is no obvious reason for the weight loss: there is no major depression, no schizophrenia, no malnutrition due to drug abuse. Examination of the patients reveals all sorts of problems in terms of their behavior and physiology. They are defensive about themselves and refuse to eat more. As a result of their starvation, there are also metabolic disturbances, including a changed blood chemistry. Because they are so sick—some may die—it is most difficult to separate the molecular abnormalities that are the result of starvation from those that may initiate the starvation. Even though some would say that these young girls are not eating because they are protesting their growth into adulthood or because they have a fear of being penetrated in any way, even by food, there is no known cause of anorexia. It is usually called a psychological disease, meaning these girls want to starve themselves rather than being compelled by something (viruses, a brain tumor, their genes, or whatever). But as is always true, the psychological can never be distinct from the physiological. In any case, there is no strong evidence that anorexia results from disturbed relationships between the sufferer and her family. In fact most disturbed family relationships produce nothing like anorexia in the children.

There is no more basic behavior to our survival than eating, and therefore it has its own control center in the brain, in a structure called the hypothalamus. An injection into this area (in rats) with a neurotransmitter molecule like norepinephrine stops even hungry rats from eating (in other brain areas we saw it caused eating). Surgical procedures in the hypothalamus of other animals can also stop eating behaviors. It is difficult to imagine that anorexia nervosa is caused by anything other than a malfunction in the eating center of the hypothalamus.

ALCOHOLISM   If you would like to take a guided tour through your evolutionary past, get off the wagon and start drinking to excess. The first drink or so of alcohol inhibits your higher brain control centers, which put restrictions on behavior. As these go out, we feel less inhibited. More drinks interfere with our thinking, as the alcohol is working its way into other brain centers, and our speech begins to slur. Soon the part of the brain that controls movement and coordination is affected and we start to wobble. Then the more primitive part of our brain controlling consciousness is knocked out. Finally, if enough alcohol is present, the oldest part of our brain, the brain stem—the first part to have evolved—is touched by the alcohol. The brain stem controls our most basic functions:

breathing and maintenance of blood pressure. When the alcohol concentration becomes high enough to inhibit the brain stem, that will be the end of the tour—you will stop breathing.

The alcoholic often drinks to a point in the above sequence where normal daily functioning is difficult or impossible. The degree of intoxication depends upon the weight of the drinker, the alcoholic content of the drink, the time over which the drinking occurs, the amount of food in the stomach, and the time of day. The effect alcohol produces depends upon the amount of alcohol in the bloodstream as it reaches the brain. The more a person weighs, the more blood there is in the body and the more diluted the alcohol becomes. To put it in other terms, a heavier person can also take a stiffer (more alcoholic) drink. If the alcohol is poured in all at once, the intoxication rate is faster because the alcohol concentration in the blood goes up faster and more alcohol reaches the brain. But if drinking goes on over a longer period of time, the body has a longer period of time to clear itself of the alcohol. With food in the stomach, alcohol molecules move less readily from the stomach into the blood, and less intoxication results. Lastly, we saw in chapter 2 that our body can tolerate more alcohol at some times of the day than at others because of biological rhythms in alcohol metabolism.

What all this is saying is that our metabolism is going to determine what alcohol does to us. Alcohol molecules are broken down and reassembled into other molecules which in turn will determine, perhaps, whether we drink in the first place, how much we drink, and whether we become dependent upon alcohol. We must not forget, however, that basically alcoholism results from drinking too much, and is cured by stopping it just as overeating is stopped by eating less. What we wish to know is why some people overdrink and do not stop.

We frequently hear that alcoholics often come from broken homes, but they come equally from unbroken homes where drinking is considered immoral. Some countries have higher alcoholism rates than others; even within a country there are differences among racial and religious groups. Such information indicates attitudes (memory molecules) toward drinking are important, because people can learn not to drink, or not to drink to excess if that is what is expected of them. Males may have a higher incidence of alcoholism than females, but why is this? Is it more acceptable for men to be drunk than for women, do they respond less well to stress than women do, are they stressed more, or is it hormonally determined? Or none of the above? Some researchers think that there are as many alcoholic women as men, but the women have been less visible to the public because they have been mostly at home. As more women enter the work force it will be interesting to see if more alcoholic women float to the surface.

Some people turn to alcohol to forget their problems, but not everyone does, even though alcohol is readily available. Taste may have a great deal of influence on drinking habits. It is known that the alcohol molecule is first broken down in the body by an enzyme into another molecule called acetaldehyde. This molecule produces quite unpleasant sensations in the body (such as nausea and headache) if allowed to accumulate and linger on without being converted by other enzymes to other types of molecules that can be excreted in the urine. In fact, the drug disulfiram is used on alcoholics to maintain a high level of acetaldehyde in the body by protecting it from being converted to other types of molecules. Therefore when alcohol is drunk, acetaldehyde accumulates and produces real discomfort to the drinker, presumably stopping further drinking. People with a metabolism that favors high acetaldehyde levels after drinking would then have a built-in protection against overdrinking. They would not have enzymes working at full efficiency to convert acetaldehyde to other molecular by-products of alcohol. Others are not so fortunate.

Some scientists speculate that the habit of alcoholism is related to internal molecular events involving acetaldehyde. One of the molecular by-products of acetaldehyde can be a substance similar in molecular structure to morphine and heroin. If the enzyme that produces this morphinelike molecule from acetaldehyde functions more effectively in some people, then these people would be expected to have a tendency to become addicted to alcohol. In one study, young men with either alcoholic parents or alcoholic siblings have been shown to have higher acetaldehyde concentrations in their blood after drinking than young men with no alcoholic parents or siblings. It would be expected that the acetaldehyde would not linger on, but would be converted into the morphinelike molecules leading to addiction. Heavy drinkers also become tolerant to alcohol, so that larger drinks are needed to achieve the same effect, just as heroin addicts need larger and larger doses.

Alcoholism may then be a matter of enzymes, all other things being equal. For some, enzymes do not get rid of acetaldehyde fast enough and the person does not like to drink much. For others, enzymes convert acetaldehyde to addictive substances and the person is hooked. As is always the case, our enzymes are products of the genes, and if there is an enzyme problem we can expect that our genes are most likely involved. Sometimes the genes may make perfect enzymes, but in order to function, the enzymes need first to attach themselves to other molecules or chemical elements such as vitamins or minerals such as magnesium. If these substances are not present in the body because of improper nutrition, the enzymes will not work. In this case it is not a genetic problem, but an enzyme-activation problem. Whatever self-improvement is necessary in overdrinking, it will have to be done by learning not to drink, because once alcohol enters the body what happens to the alcohol is going to be out of your control. Further evidence that alcoholism has a genetic basis comes from rat-breeding experiments, where strains of rats can be produced in the laboratory that seek out relatively large amounts of alcohol. A guess would be that their gene-produced enzymes are converting acetaldehyde into addictive molecules the same way our enzymes would.

The effect of acetaldehyde explains why some people do not turn to alcohol, but it does not say why others do—only that those who do turn to alcohol may have a genetic predisposition to become addicted. Some family, twin, and adoption studies suggest that some predisposition to alcoholism is inherited. We have seen some of the problems with these kinds of studies, so we have only tentative conclusions now. It has been reported, however, that the children of alcoholic parents adopted soon after birth into a nonalcoholic family showed higher rates of alcoholism than children of nonalcoholic parents adopted into other families. These adopted children of nonalcoholic parents still have lower alcoholism rates even when one of their adopted parents become alcoholic or when the parents become divorced—a source of stress. Furthermore, in the cases studied where alcoholic parents have two sons, one of which for some reason is adopted and raised by foster parents, both sons are about equally likely to become alcoholic. The significant finding here is that being *raised* by an alcoholic parent does not increase the likelihood of alcoholism in the son. The environment the son is in does not necessarily lead to his becoming alcoholic in the future. It is what he has inherited that will determine his future with alcohol. We do not know exactly what might be inherited. It may be the inability to handle stress, a tendency for compulsive behavior (an inability to quit something once started), a taste for alcohol, or an increased likelihood of addictive substances being formed after alcohol intake. As with obesity, there is no widely accepted personality profile that predicts who will be an alcoholic, so what is genetically transmitted must be rather subtle since it is not detected by psychosocial methods (written tests, interviews, recording family backgrounds, etc). The conclusion could be that if you like the taste of

alcohol, have the genes involved in converting acetaldehyde to addictive molecules, and start drinking, you will be
a genuine alcoholic regardless of what is going on around
you. One would imagine sometime in the future that these
people could take a pill with chemicals in it to destroy any
addictive molecules made by their metabolism.

HOMOSEXUALITY   Whether one considers homosexuality as an abnormality or as just an alternative life-style
depends upon how one thinks homosexuality originates.
Some people (called bisexuals or switch-hitters) engage in
both homosexual and heterosexual behavior, so it is not
necessarily a question of doing just one or the other. In
fact there is a continuum of sexual behavior ranging from
being totally heterosexual to totally homosexual. Since
performance on both fronts—or rears—is theoretically
possible by everyone, there is a wide range of desires and
behaviors directed at members of the same sex. In a few
cultures anthropologists have reported that boys practice
only homosexuality until marriage, and then drop homosexuality altogether. Since they do both, they are bisexual
and not exclusively homosexual. In other cultures homosexuality may not be that uncommon once in a while. The
same is true of heterosexual prisoners engaging in homosexuality in jails, for they return to heterosexuality when
released. Some would say that all homosexual and heterosexual behavior is learned, and that you do what the
people around you are doing. The young boys in some
cultures and some prisoners learned that it was expected
of them and that it was the only sex available. Since only
about five percent of the United States population is

estimated to be homosexual, and if learning is a factor, it must be easier to learn to be heterosexual than homosexual. If we look at the laws and attitudes against homosexuals, there certainly are impediments to learning this form of behavior. It may be just these social pressures that provoke behavioral disturbances in some homosexuals and not the homosexuality itself that produces behavioral problems.

Learning certainly plays a role in sexual attractiveness, for once experienced, one does not forget the feelings of pleasure. One can imagine, though, a man or a woman being driven away from heterosexuality by the fear of pregnancy, by a dislike of the opposite sex's body, by discouragement from participating in what others consider to be activities appropriate to their sex, or by an overprotective or seductive parent. It is usually suggested that these things produce the homosexuality, but it is equally likely that they can be the result and not the cause of a person's having homosexual feelings. Nevertheless, it is still widely believed that one's adult sexual preference is determined by one's childhood experiences and the manner in which one is raised. But there are so many ways, it is claimed, for feelings of homosexuality to begin (even in the absence of a sexual partner) that no one personality type is more likely to be homosexual than any other type. Homosexuals do not come more from one social and economic class than another, nor are there any body-build differences between homosexuals and heterosexuals. The limp-wristed, high-voiced, light-footed, hip-swinging male homosexual caricature is no more typical of a homosexual than the 6-feet-4, 250-pound male is typical of a heterosexual.

There is a strong evolutionary bias against homosexuality because it is genetically self-defeating. It is highly unlikely that there could be a prevalent gene for homosexuality, since male and female homosexuals would not wish to reproduce with each other and pass their genes on. Homosexuals face stiff competition. Some homosexuals have fathered or given birth to children, but it has not been demonstrated that their children are more likely to be homosexual than those born of heterosexual parents. If one of a pair of identical twins is homosexual, the other one is more likely to be also, than would be the case with fraternal twins if one of them were homosexual. As we have seen before, this may merely reflect similar intrauterine influences on the identical twins, or it may be the result of parents treating identical twins the same way. It is possible some say that in our evolutionary past, some degree of homosexuality was useful to the survival of the species in that those who practiced it were free of child-rearing responsibilities. This would free them to do useful things for family members engaged in raising children.

That most adults are attracted to members of the opposite sex is not questioned. Most women are attracted to something that looks like a plucked turkey neck surrounded by hair, and men are attracted to a furry hole and bumps on the chest—it must be genetic! There is good reason for this, for if the attraction were not there our species would not survive. Sex is the basic reason why we are attracted to the opposite sex. It has been suggested that sexual intercourse serves not only in reproduction but also as a way of keeping a man and woman together after childbirth, so both parents will be present to care for the young, thereby increasing the chances of survival for the offspring.

Since genes for homosexuality are not likely, and since no one can clearly point to a specific psychosocial cause, we have to look elsewhere. As indicated, there really are two kinds of homosexuals: those who always prefer sex with a member of the same sex and those who have sex with both males and females (bisexuals). As someone once remarked, there really are only two categories of people in the world anyhow: those who divide everyone up into two categories and those who do not. The discussion to follow is pertinent probably just to those men and women who are exclusively homosexual.

We know that during fetal development within the womb, molecular changes in the developing brain set patterns for sex-hormone release at puberty. There are critical periods in the intrauterine development of the organism during which the subsequent expression of sexuality may be affected if the sexual-development programs have been disrupted. The testes and ovaries of the human embryo become recognizable during the sixth week of pregnancy. This could be the start of the critical period in subsequent human sexuality, because if the testes and ovaries do not develop chemically exactly as they should, the later release of hormone molecules from these organs could be affected. The release of those hormones after puberty is under the control of the brain, which by the sixth week undergoes differentiation of its major centers. The improper development of the brain at the sixth week could also influence sex-hormone release later. The results may influence our sexual preferences at puberty and beyond. Any changes in the brain would be subtle and may only be detectable at the molecular level by chemical means.

It is currently believed that male hormones (some believe they are actually converted into estrogens before they have an effect) acting on the fetal brain of mammals during a critical period influence subsequent sexual behaviors whether the fetus is male or female. If the fetus is male and is acted upon by the male hormones, when it grows up it will exhibit masculine sexual behaviors (such as mounting females). If the fetus is female and is acted upon by the male hormones it will later exhibit some of these masculine mounting behaviors. If the male hormones do not act on the female fetus during the critical period, the grown female will act female in her sexual behavior (showing specific sexual-receptivity postures). If the male hormones do not act on the male fetus, the grown male will show fewer mounting behaviors. With humans, sexual behaviors are not as simple and clear-cut as they are for rats, mice, and guinea pigs. Male and female sexual behaviors can be much more alike in humans, so we cannot apply these animals studies directly to us. Indirectly, however, they are very suggestive of what we might expect to have an effect on our sexuality, even though all the animal sexuality studies do not always apply to us. For example, male dogs urinate differently than females do. But if female dogs are given male hormones at a certain time in the fetal stage, they will as adults assume the urinating posture of the male. I suppose we could fiddle around with these hormones during human fetal development but the subsequent costs would be enormous. We would have to reverse the signs on all men's rooms and ladies' rooms, because men would now be sitting down and women would be standing up!

Experiments with rats have demonstrated that if pregnant rats are stressed (by confinement to a small box or tube) every day for a short time during a certain critical week of their pregnancy, males born to them will not act masculine. Ninety days after birth, these males would allow themselves to be sexually mounted by other males (they would normally resist this) and would only infrequently mount female rats in heat. Stressing pregnant females at other times during gestation had essentially no effect upon their male offspring's subsequent sexual behavior. It has been found that male fetuses of stressed mother rats had different concentrations of testosterone during the critical days of brain development than did male fetuses of unstressed mothers. The interpretation: Future sexual behavior in large part is determined by how the brain develops in the fetus. It has also been shown with rats that if newborn females are injected with male hormones, they will show decreased or totally impaired receptivity to males later in life.

Female monkeys given male sex hormones during a critical time in their pregnancy give birth to females that eventually display male sexual behaviors, such as mounting other monkeys. Male hormone effects during pregnancy have also been studied in humans, in females exhibiting the adrenogenital syndrome (also called congenital adrenal hyperplasia). This is a rare genetic defect in the adrenal glands that leads to abnormalities of the genitals. The structural abnormalities are caused by an excess of male hormones acting upon the unborn fetus. If the fetus is female, behavioral effects can also be observed while the girl is growing up. Such girls act as tomboys, playing vigorous outdoor games and sports in ways that are more typical of boys. They also have little interest in playing with dolls and taking care of babies, compared to other girls. One might legitimately expect doll play and baby-care interests to be learned by watching what other girls do (and what boys do not do). It is interesting to see, though, that an overabundance of male hormones acting on the fetus can produce these behaviors when the fetus has grown up, as it were. Their more masculine behavior sets them apart from other girls of the same age because the excessive male hormones affected the molecular structure of the developing fetal brain. Treatment is available for females with the adrenogenital syndrome (since excessive male hormone levels persist) and prevents them from being masculine (deep-voiced and hairy) in appearance as adults. They are no more likely to be homosexual than any other female. The point of mentioning this syndrome is to show how prenatal influences can affect subsequent human sex-related behaviors.

We have seen from studies of mammals that a disturbance to the mother during a certain critical time of her pregnancy can markedly affect the subsequent sexual behavior of the offspring. We cannot say for sure if this is also true for humans, but it is not out of the question. We are attracted to the opposite sex because of our internal molecular structures, as we saw, and a disturbance to these brain structures during development could well eliminate it or redirect the attractiveness to the same sex. What the disturbances might be which would affect sex-hormone levels in the fetal brain is not known. They may be the mother's diet, infections, drugs, stress, or random intrauterine events. After puberty the sex hormones have no effect on sexual preference when injected into humans. For instance, female hormones (estrogens) do not make male homosexuals more homosexual, nor do male hormones (testosterones) make them less homosexual. Injected male hormones also have no effect upon the sexual behavior of human female homosexuals.

There is some slight evidence that human male homosexuals may have lower testosterone levels in their body than male heterosexuals do, and that bisexual males have testosterone levels midway between homosexuals and heterosexuals. In addition, human female homosexuals may have higher testosterone levels than heterosexual females. Since it is also known that male soldiers starting basic training and those about to leave on a combat mission also have lower-than-average testosterone levels, we may have to conclude that stress is the cause and not homosexuality. The lower levels for homosexuals may be the result of stress they are subjected to by society's pressures to conform.

Masters and Johnson, the American sex researchers, claim those homosexuals who are motivated to change their sexual life-style can be helped by psychotherapy. Such conversational therapy concentrates not on the causes of their homosexuality, but on the problems a homosexual life-style has created for them. Those who wish to change may be just those who have learned their type of sexual preferences; psychotherapy helps them unlearn it. Their first sexual experiences may have been homosexual and they learned to like it. They may have preferred heterosexuality but could not obtain it, so they satisfied their sexual needs with a homosexual who was available. They may have had bad heterosexual experiences and turned to homosexuality as the next best thing.

In contrast to this group there are homosexuals who have no desire to change. Their sexual preferences may have been ultimately determined by intrauterine stress events and have nothing at all to do with learning this behavior. Consequently, there would be nothing to unlearn by psychotherapy and it would be totally ineffective. These homosexuals would think of their behavior as perfectly normal, and for them it would be.

OBESITY, ALCOHOLISM, AND HOMOSEXUALITY

We need only to look to find an alcoholic, homosexual, or an obese person. We can readily see that they exist and are not imaginary, yet we cannot psychologically characterize the type of person who is likely to become any one of these—although not for lack of trying. Behavioral scientists have been intensively studying these behaviors for a long time and we still know very little about their psychosocial development. It is tempting to conclude that this is because the psychosocial factors are secondary to the physiological ones. The physiological or molecular basis of these behaviors has been studied by fewer researchers over a shorter period of time with more suggestive results, which indicate that metabolic factors are of prime importance in alcoholism and obesity, and intrauterine ones appear to be important in homosexuality. Add to this whatever the psychosocial environment contributes, and we will obtain a good preliminary understanding of the origin of these behaviors. Obesity, alcoholism, and homosexuality can be stopped quite simply, it would appear, by not doing them anymore. We cannot simply stop being a schizophrenic or a manic-depressive. But as it turns out, we really cannot stop being obese, alcoholic, or homosexual that easily, as anybody knows who has tried. The reason: These behaviors, like all others, are generated by the molecules within, working in predetermined patterns not easily modified by intentions.

STRESS   If we define stress as the psychosocial and physical forces acting upon us, then stress cannot be avoided. Indeed, the only escape from stress is death. Physically we are subjected to temperature, light, and humidity changes that our bodies must adjust to, and to pollutants in air, water, and food that our bodies must handle. We must also confront the behavioral expectations of others, and the financial and sexual demands upon our life. With stress such a part of our life, it is not surprising that we think it should cause many of our problems, such as alcoholism, obesity, aggression, schizophrenia, mania-depression, and such things as heart disease and maybe even cancer. In all these cases, however, the evidence that stress alone produces their onset is not strong. In fact, the correlation between stress of a psychosocial nature (family and job pressures, for example) and physical illness of any sort is not great. Most stress studies have been initiated after an illness has been detected. If patients, doctors, and researchers think stress is responsible for the illness, then they will find some previous stressful event to prove they were right. They have self-fulfilling expectations. Stress may more likely be the result of the illness and not the cause. The amount of stress people have been subjected to has been measured and it does not predict very well at all the likelihood of subsequent accidents or illnesses, whether they be minor medical complaints or more serious ones like leukemia, heart attack, diabetes, or multiple sclerosis. While some people with these medical problems have been subjected to higher stress levels in the course of their lives, others subjected to higher stress levels did not develop these illnesses.

      This is not to say stress never has an effect on us. It does, but it does not seem to produce medical illnesses for most of us. Stress can affect our behavior, however. For example, many individuals find it difficult to work under pressure. This means that they cannot concentrate on their work because they are thinking about the consequences of their work and not about the work itself. The athlete who chokes under pressure (stress) is not concentrating on throwing the ball or hitting it or catching it, but is diverting attention to thinking about what will happen to his or her career or image if it is done badly, or the rewards if done well.

      It is said that the friends and relatives close to us, the amount of money we have, our education, and previous experiences with stress can help us manage stress. If we have been through it before, we can better handle repeated stress, unless the stress was so bad the first time that we could not bear to undergo it again. Financial losses are better sustained if you still have adequate funds left, but even so, some wealthy people are stressed by the losses, while some without funds do not worry about it. Supportive friends and relatives sometimes are a help and sometimes not. The prediction is that an educated, financially well-off person, subjected to stresses experienced before and aided by friends and relatives is not likely to be affected by stress. How can we be sure? Even in the absence of these factors, one may still not be affected by stress. As another example, not all children of divorced parents suffer behaviorally from this stress. On the other hand, the death of one's child or spouse is stressful enough to affect virtually everyone. Similarly, the concentration and prisoner-of-war camps of Germany and Japan in World War II produced so much stress that virtually everyone there showed changes in behavior. When the stress is less, the relationship of stress to changes in behavior is not so predictable given only information about the social situation. What is needed is molecular information.

After our senses take in psychosocial information from our environment and convert it into molecular information to feed to the brain, the brain decides whether the environmental events are stressful or not. Now the past experiences and present situation of the individual come into play. One remembers whether one has previously experienced this stress and what its outcome was, so one can evaluate the seriousness of the stress. Other facts come out of memory to be evaluated by a decision-making process: Will one's knowledge, finances, or friends be able to help? If the right facts do not come out of memory at the right time, a less than optimal evaluation of the stressful event will occur. On the other hand, if this stress never occurred before, there is no way to predetermine the best course of action. This is why we cannot predict very well what any given person will do in response to most stresses—we do not know how the brain is assessing the stress.

On the other hand, given that stress-producing factors are present, we can trace some of the molecular events that are produced. One well-known physiological reaction to stress is the fight-or-flight response. It is the same response we have when we get stage fright. This occurs when the stress is such that we either fear the situation and wish to escape from it (flight), or wish to stand our ground and fight. Information about the situation reaches our brain and may trigger the fight-or-flight response by releasing adrenaline molecules into our bloodstream. The adrenaline increases our breathing rate so that more oxygen molecules are available, and it increases our heart rate to speed up the circulation of this oxygen to our muscles, which need it to help us move. At the same time, the blood circulation is reduced to our internal organs like the stomach, since the immediate need for blood and its nutrients is to help the muscles move our arms and legs to help us fight or run away. Some of the fat in our body is broken down into simpler molecules as a source of energy for our muscular activity (see Figure 11). In addition, molecular events take place in our blood that allow it to coagulate more readily than usual, should we bleed from an injury during fighting. We may also sweat and shake a little. All these events result from stress to the body and are not a cause of it.

There is also a more general physiological response to stress called the general adaptation syndrome or the biological stress syndrome. The initial molecular response to stress is pretty much the same regardless of whether the stress is caused by temperature extremes to the body, pain, fear, surgery, or anxiety. Stress from fasting and severe exercise do not seem to produce the same responses, though. All of these stressors (and many other ones) cause the release of hydrocortisone (also called cortisol) molecules into the bloodstream. What happens is this: All sensory information about the world around us can be delivered by nerve impulses to a region of the brain called the hypothalamus. If these impulses carry a stressful message, the hypothalamus secretes molecules which cause another portion of the brain, the pituitary, to release ACTH (adrenocorticotrophic hormone) molecules into the bloodstream. Presumably the hypothalamus will recognize as stressful only those nerve impulses with specific chemical and physical properties that have been programmed into the brain. The ACTH molecules reach our adrenal glands (located on top of our kidneys) and cause them to secrete hydrocortisone into the bloodstream. Increased hydrocortisone levels have been measured in humans anticipating new or unpleasant situations (such as surgery or college examinations), airplane flights, and during certain jobs and athletic competitions.

Once the hydrocortisone is in our bloodstream, it ends up in all parts of the body, just as any other chemical in the blood does. However, not all cells respond to all chemicals. Every one of our cells has certain specific receptor sites on its surface that bind or hold onto only certain specific molecules when they touch the cell. Consequently, male sex-hormone molecules circulating in the bloodstream could bind to skin cells to promote hair growth in men, but could not bind to stomach or liver cells where they have no function. Similarly, hydrocortisone binds only to certain cells, and the location of the cells in our body determines the effect. We do know some of the things hydrocortisone does. Some protein molecules in certain cells are broken down into their constituent amino acids, and some are reassembled in a multistep process into sugars to serve as an energy source (see Figure 11 again) during the stress. The remaining amino acids can be used to synthesize proteins that may have been destroyed in tissue damage resulting from the stress. Tissue damage also causes inflammation, which is combated by the hydrocortisone released during the stress syndrome. While tissue damage may not result from the stress, nor increased energy supplies be needed, the body is preparing itself just in case fighting and injury result. This does say something about aggression being a part of our life, since the body is anticipating it!

The different ways different people react to stress can be understood in terms of the biological-stress syndrome we have been discussing. The hypothalamus brain program that recognizes stress when it comes in over the nerves is certainly a source of variability. Some people may feel stressed when not much has happened to them; they have a low tolerance for stress. For others it may take considerably more stress before the hypothalamus identifies it as such; these people have a high tolerance for stress. Once the hydrocortisone is released by the adrenals, however, there could also be variability from person to person in the cell's response to it. Some cells may detect it more readily than others. So the molecular structure of our hypothalamus, and the degree to which our cells respond to hydrocortisone, may be the main source of variability in our responses to stress. Some people will feel stress more because more is happening chemically in their body. It is likely that hydrocortisone and other molecules released during stress have many other effects upon the body besides combating possible tissue damage. When we find out more about this we may have a clearer picture of the true relationship of stress to heart disease, alcoholism, obesity, and some forms of mental illness.

HAPPINESS We know more about what makes a rat happy than ourselves. Over twenty years ago a pleasure center in a rat's brain was discovered. By sending an electric current through a thin wire inserted into the brain, a rat could be made exquisitely happy. If given a choice of food or the electrical stimulation, the rat would choose (or its brain would choose for it) the electrical stimulation. It was subsequently found that rats would go to great lengths to obtain this stimulation, ignoring food to the point of starvation and ignoring sleep to the point of exhaustion. We know from our own experience that when we are doing something we very much like, something very pleasurable, we do not get hungry or tired, although we stop short of starvation. Not every part of the brain can be stimulated to produce this pleasure. In fact, some locations of the brain, upon being electrically stimulated, force the rat to try to escape such stimulation. It is a particular site in the hypothalamus region of the brain, though, that gives the most pleasure when stimulated. Interestingly, these brain pleasure centers have also been found in fish, birds, and monkeys. In view of our close evolutionary relationship to monkeys, we should have such pleasure centers also.

We do not know how these centers really function, but there is evidence that pleasure involves the participation of the molecule dopamine, another neurotransmitter chemical found in brains. Drugs like the amphetamines (which facilitate the action of dopamine in certain nerve cells in the hypothalamus) increase the rate at which rats seek out the stimulation. Amphetamines may elevate our moods and give us feelings of pleasure by enhancing dopamine action in our brain. Other drugs—like reserpine and chlorpromazine, which interfere with the action of dopamine molecules—decrease the rate at which stimulation for pleasure is sought.

These brain pleasure centers do not exist just to be electrically stimulated by scientists, who after all did not come onto the scene for millions of years after the rat was already here and happy. When these centers are turned on by what the organism is doing, it is happy; this may be the real meaning of being "turned on." A guess would be that when certain nerves are activated by the behaviors of sexual activity, eating and drinking, creative thinking, listening to music, jogging, or whatever, special nerve signals are sent along those nerves to the hypothalamus pleasure center. This action informs us that we are happy. In other words, a specific, well-defined pattern of incoming nerve signals has to occur before the brain interprets the triggering activity as pleasurable. All other things being equal (we are not comparing the poor with the rich, the handicapped with the gifted, etc.), the differences among people in how happy they are may well reflect differences in how the pleasure center of the hypothalamus functions.

Differences in happiness may also be reflected by how many endorphin molecules we have in certain brain centers. As naturally occurring brain opiates, the endorphins function as internal painkillers and produce euphoria just like the opiates morphine and heroin. Those with more endorphins released with certain activities may be happier about any given situation or event in their lives than those with fewer endorphins. That is, doing the same thing may be more pleasurable to one person than another because for that person, more endorphin molecules are released in the brain. Happiness, then, lies not outside the body, but within. Happiness is not an illusion; it is real and has a molecular basis. We might ask why we should be happy. Why should our brain have happiness centers and happiness chemicals? It may be that happiness or pleasure makes life worth living so that we will want to live long enough to reproduce and care for our young until they reach a reproductive age. The avoidance of grief also makes life more pleasant. Knowing how painful it is may make us avoid grief as long as possible by protecting and caring for those closest to us. Grief serves to have us care more. This is another indication that some of our behaviors are designed to perpetuate the species.

PERSONALITY   If personality is defined as the total of the observable behaviors of a person, then all the behaviors discussed so far contribute to our personality. There are many other aspects of our personality as well. Many of these are measured by administering written psychological tests. These tests measure such personality traits as trustfulness, independence, responsibility, and flexibility. These tests are quite reliable in that if one takes the test again, one obtains pretty much the same results. However, what the tests measure relative to underlying physiological processes is uncertain. For example, questions in a personality test can ask to what degree you trust your spouse, friends, neighbors, relatives, coworkers, strangers, etc. From the answers one could get a relative idea of how trustful any given person is, and call it a trustful personality trait. This kind of trait would seem to be learned and would be based on the experiences one had in trusting others.

Another personality trait such as self-control may have very little to do with learning experiences. Self-control may reflect how our higher brain centers are wired up to control our lower brain centers that initiate aggression and emotional outbursts such as anger and crying. Thus, we are born with some personality traits that do not change very much throughout our lives. Other traits are very much influenced by the psychosocial environment. It is often observed that people, as they approach old age, become more childlike in their personality. It is as though the personality traits which they acquired through a lifetime of learning and which made them mature are forgotten or cast aside. What remains are the personality traits they were born with, the ones most noticeable in children before they learn fully what their culture has to teach them.

All personality traits represent a mixture of many physiological processes that have not yet been sorted out. Personality factors therefore have no specific biological meaning—they are constructed without reference to any biological structure or process. As with the concept of intelligence, personality traits did not exist in nature until they were measured. In any case, personality tests measure something about our behavior even though it is seldom obvious what the biological basis of it is. Where these tests have been given to identical and fraternal twins, the identical twins usually show closer personality traits (similar behaviors) than fraternal twins do. More importantly, identical twins raised apart from one another still have several similar personality traits. These are the traits most dependent upon genetic influences, like self-control. Other personality traits are much more influenced by the environment, like trustfulness.

Studies with human infants have revealed that some of the personality traits observed at two months of age can also be observed when the children have reached ten years. For instance, infants who are constantly moving around (even during sleep), are easily distracted, and who have short attention spans are found at ten years to be those children who cannot sit still for very long and need a very quiet environment when doing their homework. The results of these studies show that children exhibit certain personality traits before their parents can interact very much with them. Studies with newborns have demonstrated that minor physical defects (such as malformed ears, a curved fifth finger, an abnormal distance between the eyes or ears, more than one hair whorl on the scalp, plus twelve other measures) are correlated with hyperactivity (short attention span, overactivity, impulsiveness, excitability) at age three. While many of us may have two or three of these "defects," an excess number of them reflects more serious underlying abnormalities that occurred during the development of the fetus. It is thought some insult to the fetus may have occurred during pregnancy that disrupted the normal development of the baby, producing both hyperactivity and these minor physical defects.

There is evidence (disputed by some) hyperactivity is elicited by substances in the diet of children. The substances thought to have an effect are certain artificial food dyes which may increase neurotransmitter release in the nervous system. As we saw in chapter 4 with mania, increased numbers of neurotransmitter molecules can lead to increased behavioral activity, because nerve impulses are moving more quickly in the body. When hyperactive children are placed on a diet free from artificial food dyes, about half of them show a decrease in hyperactivity. Futhermore, giving food dyes to hyperactive children (who for three previous days were kept off them in their diets) causes them to shorten their attention span and to do less well on tests of learning ability. Giving these same dyes to children of the same age and sex who were never diagnosed as hyperactive produced no changes in behavior. The dyes exerted their effects on the hyperactive

children within one and one-half hours and lasted at least
for three and one-half hours. Such fast action is typical of
a drug effect. Any number of psychosocial theories
implicating inadequate family and school situations could
be proposed to explain how hyperactivity develops in the
child. But as I have explained, these theories are always
very difficult to support because the real proof is to
remove the children from the faulty environment and see
if the behavior goes away. Then put them back in it and
see if the hyperactive behavior returns. Such manipulations of the child relative to his or her environment is
seldom possible as it involves changing schools, friends, or
the family. In contrast, see how relatively simple it was to
show a chemical effect: Take the food-dye chemicals away
and hyperactivity goes away. Add the food-dye chemicals
back to the diet and hyperactivity returns. A chemical
might not have an effect, but that too is relatively easy to
establish. By no means do these dye experiments wrap up
the problem of hyperactivity, since not every hyperactive
child was affected by the dyes, and not all the possible
hyperactive behaviors were produced by the dyes. The
dyes would appear to turn on hyperactive behavior in
those children who already had the molecular brain
structure to predispose them to hyperactivity.

Studies have shown that women given progestin
and estrogen sex hormones during pregnancy (to prevent
miscarriages) gave birth to children that subsequently
showed modified personalities. To be sure, the children's
personalities were not abnormal, just altered. Compared
to children of mothers receiving no hormonal treatment
during pregnancy, they showed differences upon testing

in their self-assertiveness and independence. It is not known whether these personality changes would accompany the children into adulthood. We saw that changes in prenatal sex-hormone levels could affect fetal brain development and produce subsequent behavioral changes in aggression and sexual behavior. It is not too surprising, therefore, to find some elements of personality being affected by increased sex-hormone levels moving into the fetal brain across the placenta. It is known that children born to heroin-addicted mothers tend to be more irritable and hyperactive than other children. However, a variety of drugs have been used on these children to help them through heroin withdrawal (if the mother is addicted, so is the fetus), and these drugs may be producing the behavioral changes. In addition, heroin addicts have poor nutritional habits and often use other drugs (nicotine, barbiturates, alcohol) to excess. These offer further insults to the developing fetal brain. Regardless of which of the many drugs might be affecting the unborn, the fact is that personality can be altered by interfering with the molecular development of the brain.

A child's behavior can also be changed by exposure to chemicals in the environment. Long-term exposure to low concentrations of lead molecules has been shown to affect the classroom performance of children. They performed less well than others not exposed to lead in terms of their attention, concentration, and organization of schoolwork. They also showed some deficits in their speech and in understanding directions, but in no case did they have high enough lead concentrations to be considered lead poisoned. These were not hereditary problems,

211

nor were these behavioral changes related to the parents' socioeconomic status, a bad family situation, or nutritional problems. The effect was purely (or impurely) environmental, though it was the physical and not the psychosocial environment that was involved. They were learning disabled because of long-term exposure to low concentrations of lead that affected brain function. The amount of lead in a child's body was directly related to his or her classroom difficulty. The source of the lead could have been from batteries, paints, certain kinds of ceramic dishes, and/or from the air (most of the lead in the air is from vehicles using leaded gasoline).

Of all the effects upon our personality, none is more pervasive than our temperament, our overall emotional response. It is something we are born with and have with us throughout our life whether we be human, dog, horse, or whatever. We have to be high enough on the evolutionary scale to have enough variability in behavior to produce a temperament as one never sees a nervous sponge or a reckless sea urchin, for example. Temperament is our disposition, our emotional makeup, and our manner of behavior, which affects all that we do. There are any number of ways to categorize temperament, such as saying someone is nervous versus calm, pleasant versus unpleasant, flexible versus inflexible, cautious versus reckless, and so on. Each of these descriptions applies in different degrees to all of us. Temperament is essentially the sum of everything that is our personality. It is the bottom line, so to speak, on our behavior. What the corresponding biological entities are that produce temperament is not known. In a general sense it depends upon how our brain is wired, that is, upon what nerve-impulse pathways we have and how they function at the molecular level. Whatever it is that generates our temperament, it is isolated from the outside world, as it seldom changes. Our outward-directed temperament reflects inner biology.

Another aspect of our personality that seems to reflect inner biological processes is the introversion-extroversion personality factor. This is a composite of behaviors that measures to what extent we are sociable and outgoing (extroversion) or tend to keep to ourselves (introversion). It is thought that introversion-extroversion is determined by the arousal center of our brain. If this center is not activated, then we are not going to be alert, or even very much awake. In some unknown way, introverts are self-starting and activate this center from within. Extroverts, on the other hand, must depend mainly upon outside social contacts to activate their center. The extrovert keeps his or her brain lively by interacting with people. The introvert can do this without social contact. Most likely, which one we are is established by the time we are born.

One cannot help but wonder about what unknown molecular influences have shaped our adult lives, working their magic independently of the psychological and social forces around us. The conclusion from these studies is that we are born with some personality traits, like temperament, self-control, and introversion-extroversion. Other traits can be modified by lead, food dyes, and sex hormones. As research continues, it will be interesting to find out what other behaviors are present at birth and to what extent personalities can be modified by both the chemical and psychosocial environment.

If a body is not quite right molecularly, self-improvement becomes that much more difficult. If the developing fetus is stressed in some way, it can be delivered at birth with personality traits that will be with it perhaps for life, and with even a tendency for homosexual behavior after puberty. Having enzyme molecules in the body that attack food and alcohol molecules in peculiar ways can lead to obesity and alcoholism. Brain chemicals can determine how happy we are likely to be. We all know it is not easy to change fundamental aspects of our behavior, and now we know why. It is difficult to get our molecular act together.

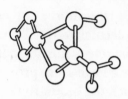

Molecular Bondage

Ultimately, behavior depends upon just one thing: molecules—which ones we have and where they are at any given time within our body. Which ones we have is a matter of genetics and nutrition. Nutrition provides the raw materials for building molecules, and our genes direct the assembly of molecules. From the moment an egg and a sperm fuse to initiate the formation of the human embryo we are dependent upon the proper nutritional environment to supply us with the necessary molecules to use directly or to reassemble for growth and maintenance. Where the molecules are depends upon how freely molecules can move around in our body. The structure of our cells and tissues allows some molecules and atoms to move freely in or out and restricts the passage of others. Our cells are constructed to allow molecules to move from the site of synthesis or assembly to the site of use. Cells also allow nutrients to enter and waste products to leave.

Chance also plays a role in determining where our molecules are, because our body heat bounces molecules about at random. Furthermore, our environment influences where our molecules move. Events in the environment that activate our senses initiate molecular and atomic movements that, as we have seen, produce nerve impulses which eventually reach the brain. In response to them, the brain can produce other nerve impulses to communicate with other parts of the body, which may respond by moving molecules around also. For example, we see something; nerve impulses are initiated by the eyes. The impulses reach the brain which, let us say, interprets what we have seen as frightening. Nerve impulses are then sent to the adrenal glands located over the kidneys. The adrenal glands allow adrenaline molecules to move into the bloodstream, eventually affecting, among other things, our rate of breathing. (You will recall from the previous chapter that this is the fight-or-flight response.) Our breathing rate in turn determines how many oxygen molecules move into our lungs. Clearly the environment rearranges our molecules, but within limits set by our physiology.

INSIDE AND OUTSIDE INFLUENCES   An illustration of how our behavior is determined can be found in Figure 12. The environment—the world outside our body—can influence our behavior by getting into our brain directly through our senses, or by entering another part of our body. The people we interact with, the things we hear, the places we visit, and the events we experience enter through our senses. They may become a part of our ongoing physiology and affect our behavior. For instance, we witness an automobile accident, and what we see and hear is converted into molecular events by our senses. They are stored in our brain by physiological processes in the brain. Then the memory of the accident reminds us to be more careful in our driving. Although, as we saw in chapter 3 in discussing memory, most of what our senses take in has no effect upon our behavior. In driving to work, most of the buildings, trees, people, and things we pass will not affect us in any way. We saw in chapter 4 that virus infections could modify our behavior, but as micro-organisms they might not enter our body through the senses. Other viruses that get in may have no effect.

Events generated inside the person can also affect behavior. Random events and genetic influences within the body modify behavior, as Figure 12 demonstrates. Chance is difficult to handle because if something happens by chance, we mean it is unpredictable. When we flip a coin the outcome is either heads or tails, and we cannot predict which it will be—either is equally likely. With the trillions of trillions of molecules in our body bouncing around, there will always be some chance that the right molecules will not be at the right place at the right time. Since our behavior depends upon molecules being at the right locations, disturbances can change our behavior. Chance has no feelings, so we cannot blame its effects on anyone. The extent to which chance molecular events influence our thinking was discussed in chapter 3. But chance plays a role in most of our behaviors. By chance, we may be in an environment that triggers a behavior. We walk down one street and nothing happens; but we walk down another one and we are mugged, so we fight back. By chance, in our development in the womb, molecules moved this way or that in our brain and we end up homosexual, or bad tempered.

Our genes also have an effect upon our behavior. They set the limits on what we can do and what our senses can take in, while internal chance events and the environment determine just how close we can come to the limits. If you were born with a potentially poor singing voice (physiology and genes), all the lucky career breaks (chance) and training (environmental influence) will not help with a singing career. But if the genes give you that rare molecular combination of a voice box and musical brain center, your voice still will not reach its potential without input from the environment (training).

If you believe this, is it too much to accept the thought that not everyone is born with the potential to be intelligent? No one seems to think we can turn every adult male into a professional football player, where the important factors of physical size, aggressiveness, coordination, and quickness have at least some relationship to genetics. The best athletic-training environment will not help the small-boned, mild-mannered, uncoordinated male make the team. It may be that everyone cannot be educated to be intelligent either. But you say singing and football are physical, not mental, and it is not the same as being intelligent. Such a distinction is not justified since, as I argued in chapter 1, mind and body cannot be separated. Both depend upon molecules for their existence. We have

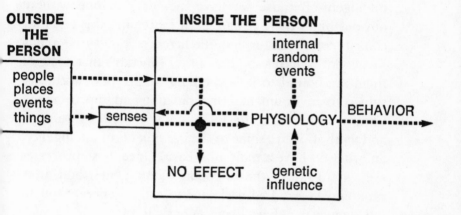

Figure 12: DETERMINATION OF BEHAVIOR
If something outside our body is to influence our behavior, it must first get inside our body in some form. Then the outside influences can interact with our genetics, physiology, and random events to produce a behavior. Some things may get inside the body but still have no effect. Internal events may also affect our senses.

seen some of the problems in properly defining what intelligence really is, so we speak of it in relative terms: Someone is more intelligent than someone else, or less intelligent. Because we have memory, anyone without obvious brain damage can learn more, and this certainly contributes to his or her intelligence. But to be really intelligent requires so many brain functions that some of them are bound to be something we are born with, not subject to environmental manipulation and improvement. Creativity, thinking, decision making, memory storage, and motivation are some of the ingredients of intelligence, and they all have a molecular basis. Once these processes are set up under the direction of the genes, and after randomness has had a chance to act, a general limit to intelligence may have been set early in life.

THE NATURE OF NURTURE   If nature means the contribution of genes to behavior, and nurture means the contribution of the environment—all outside influences —then a nature-nurture argument would be over the relative contribution of each. We have seen that both are important, but sometimes one is more important than another. Including the contribution of chance, we can say that in practice:

$$100\% \text{ Behavior} = X\% \text{ Genes} + Y\% \text{ Environmental Influence} + Z\% \text{ Chance}$$

Since genes (and the physiology they direct), environmental influences (including of course what we learn from our culture), and chance are the only causes of behavior, $X\%$ + $Y\%$ + $Z\%$ must equal 100% (or all) of behavior. The evidence presented in this book suggests not only that these three components do not contribute equally to behavior, but also that the relative contribution of the three components varies from one behavior to another. It is not sufficient to say that genes and the environment contribute equally. That is, it would be incorrect to say that 100% behavior = 50% genes + 50% environment, not only because the element of chance is disregarded, but also because the relative importance of genes to environment varies from behavior to behavior. At present, we just do not know enough to give accurate numbers for X, Y, and Z in the equation, but the best current guess is that they are not equal.

This book, besides indicating the molecular nature of behavior, has called into question the relative importance of the psychosocial environment for some behaviors. No one can dismiss the environment entirely as an influence, but its relative importance in determining some behaviors can be questioned. There are two reasons for this. First, biological studies are showing that some important behaviors develop primarily because of internal physiological events, with psychosocial events assuming secondary importance. We have seen these internal processes at work in producing mental illness, the tendency to love and hate, and in inhibiting molecular self-improvement. Second, there is not objective proof that the psychosocial environment causes many of the behaviors discussed in this book. The reason for this is simple. We cannot manipulate people into two experimental groups, with each receiving different psychosocial experiences, during their development into adulthood to see which group gets damaged by interactions with the environment and which does not. It must be clear that there is no proof of this kind for arguments emphasizing the physiological causes of behavior either. With few exceptions (generalized anxiety disorder in chapter 4 and hyperactivity in chapter 6) we cannot inject chemicals into people to see what damages or changes their behavior. These two reasons for questioning the environment indicate that we must now consider both the physiological and psychosocial causes of behavior. As we learn more about behavior, we can determine which of the two influences our molecules the most, as well as properly assessing the role of chance.

ESCAPE FROM BONDAGE The chemical bonds that bind our molecules together, in turn bind us to the past. We cannot ignore the three billion years of evolution that produced the human species and that make us function on a molecular level. We are the product of a continuing series of molecular rearrangements over the course of evolution that up until now we could do little about. But of all the living things, we are most able to modify our behavior by willing it to change. We are not always obliged to give the same response to the same stimulus as are our animal predecessors, since we have a wider range of responses at our disposal. This flexibility is due to an increased memory and thinking capacity in our brain. It is this kind of flexibility that lets us control our aggression and love better than animals probably do. On the other hand, the freedom to respond to some situations in a variety of ways may create a decision-making stress that may be related to a variety of unwanted behaviors including, perhaps, mental illness. This does not mean that we can consciously modify all our behaviors to control our responses with regard to overeating, alcohol, sex, and aggression, or that we can think our way out of mental illness or biological rhythms. Some behaviors may be locked in more than we would like, while others may be quite modifiable.

Heredity predetermines everything up to a point, since it determines our potential, but the expression of this potential can be modified by any number of things. Heredity we know is not necessarily destiny. As Figure 12 illustrates, both chance and the environment interact with our genes to produce our behavior. In other words, the expression of genes (the molecules they produce) can be interfered with, and so our behavior can be modified. Some possible modifiers of gene expression that have been mentioned in this book are: parental and intrauterine influences, stress, learning, interpersonal relationships, time of day (biorhythms), nutritional deficits, and infection with microorganisms. In terms of Figure 12, these modifiers come from the people, places, things, and events around us. The degree to which they modify gene expression determines to what extent we can escape our heredity. If we can significantly modify our behavior through learning, by changing child-rearing practices, by removing stress, by proper nutrition and disease prevention, then we can change our destiny by changing our behavior. If not, then we have to go where our molecules take us without much prospect of fighting back except at the molecular level. The bad thing about genes determining our behavior is that an untalented person would not be helped much by a change to a more favorable environment. The good thing is that a very talented person would not be hurt much by an unfavorable environment. Most people are neither very untalented nor very talented, and for them the environment is going to be much more an important influence in today's world. Of course if we are talking about extreme environmental conditions such as the presence of slavery or famine, or armed oppression, then no one, no matter how talented, can get out.

Only the briefest look back into history tells us that our culture—how we live—is different from what it once was. But we are living differently now because we have learned to do so and have passed our learning on to subsequent generations, and not because our internal molecular structures have changed. They, in fact, have probably not changed for the past forty thousand years or so. That is, we are probably the same, genetically, now as we were forty thousand years ago when our species (*Homo sapiens sapiens*) evolved into its present form. Without doubt we are the same genetically now as we were about ten thousand years ago when the first villages were built in the Middle East. We have no new kinds of genes since then. If all our recorded history were destroyed (including books, newspapers, magazines, documents, notes, microfilms, computer tapes, photos, etc.) and our memory somehow erased, it could take us again about ten thousand years or maybe forty thousand years to get back to where we are now, more or less. We cannot discount the role of chance in history, so it is very unlikely we would be exactly where we are today. Consider just one invention, the airplane, as an example of how our basic thinking has not changed. The Egyptians of four thousand years ago, the

Greeks of twenty-five hundred years ago, and the Europeans of one thousand years ago failed to build airplanes not because their brains were incapable of complex thought —their brains were as capable of it as ours. They failed because they had not yet learned about the factors contributing to manned flight. They had not accumulated enough information to put it all together. They had not invented an engine small enough and powerful enough, nor did they have a high-energy fuel like gasoline. Besides, where were they going to fly to? They might go off the edge of the earth. While they built boats of wood, they did not use wood to make lightweight manned gliders to study how heavier-than-air objects could fly. Possibly the thought of a person flying was objectional to them on religious grounds. But bit by bit we gathered enough information to learn to fly, and we have learned that no curse will befall us for flying, except perhaps an occasional crash to remind us that we are terrestrial animals.

If our genes have not changed for at least ten thousand years, then we might expect that there would be no fundamental change in our behavior either over this time period. We have learned to do different things, such as develop assembly lines and run our governments, but the molecular components in our brain that produce the learning and the thinking have not changed and could not change unless our genes had changed. The molecular structures that allow aggression, love, obesity, alcoholism, homosexuality, creativity, and mental illness to exist are the same now as they were ten thousand years ago. As our environment and culture have changed, new situations arose, but the basic responses were built in before ten thousand years ago. Perhaps our destiny was really set down then. If we are any better behaved now, it is not because we are genetically better. It is because we have learned to be better.

MYTH AND REALITY   The laws, values, ethics, and morals that we have developed over the past five thousand years of recorded history eventually reflect what we know about our own biology. They are slowly but continually being readjusted to take account of new knowledge about nature, and in this sense stand between man and nature. If you will, knowledge about our physiology gives us some clues in our search for rules and principles to live by. People stopped accusing others of using witchcraft and trying them as witches as they began to believe the world was governed by more natural processes (reality) than by superstition (myth). On the other hand, slavery was outlawed in the Western world before we had any solid biological evidence that all races are of the same species (although some did suspect this), with no race being superior to any other one. In fact, the end to slavery may have been brought about partly because of the availability of machines to do the work of slaves. Only relatively recently have we seen that all races have evolved from a common ancestor, and that we all share a common molecular structure. With this biological knowledge, the world will never again tolerate slavery. It does occur in isolated instances, but its presence when revealed will produce a worldwide outcry. However, we still torture people because we learned long ago that there is a strong biological drive to avoid pain. To avoid it we will "confess" and open up our memory to others. While torture may be illegal and provoke an outcry, it certainly has not disappeared to the extent slavery has, and it will not, because it has a biological basis for working.

Clearly, getting closer to our biological self is not always what we would hope for. There is no guarantee we will like what we are. When we know what our genes are and what they are capable of doing, then we can get closer to what we can expect of ourselves. What happens to our freedom? Are we now freer because we know our limitations? If we know the rules of the game, we are freer to deal with the realities of that game. But our freedom to persist in myth will be curtailed. If we know exactly what we have to work with, we can start to work with it that much more quickly. It may be much easier for us to believe in myth than in reality because there are no limits to where myth can take us. Reality ties us down and forces us to deal directly with the problems and prospects we have, and stops us from looking for excuses or help that does not exist.

Presently, the predominant thinking is that the psychosocial environment has caused most of our behavioral problems, and we treat the problems accordingly: We blame the societies that produced them. When we realize that many behaviors depend less upon the psychosocial environment and more upon internal molecular activities, we can stop looking for someone to blame. We can get down to dealing with the problem at the molecular level. We do not hold other people to blame for someone else's kidney failure, stroke, cataracts, or epilepsy. Why must we always blame someone for another person's mental illness, alcoholism, obesity, aggression, or personality? Would it not be better for parents to know that their interactions with their child did not cause hyperactivity, learning disorders, or homosexuality? Would they not be freer of guilt and doubt? Once we get used to it, reality may be much easier to live with than myth. Even for those behaviors that are strongly influenced by what is happening around us, we must acknowledge that our physiology will still determine our response.

REDUCTIONISM   There is no doubt that I am saying we can reduce all our behaviors down to the action of molecules and atoms. This is called reductionism. The point of reductionism is to give us the ultimate explanation of why we do what we do. Not everyone believes in reductionism—some say there is more to life than just atoms and molecules. (Of course, there is not!) If we only study these, the argument goes, we will miss the vital force that makes it all work. It has been said that reductionists learn more and more about less and less until they know everything about nothing. It could be said of the antire-ductionists that they learn less and less about more and more until they know nothing about everything. Some fear that if we reduce behavior down too far, the behavior will have no meaning, because the whole is greater or different than the sum of its parts. A word has no meaning when reduced to its separate letters standing alone. Similarly, when we investigate such behaviors as love and hate, we realize that there will be no such things as love molecules or hate molecules. These behaviors are pro-duced by enormous numbers of different kinds of molecules interacting with each other. Behavior has no meaning when just one or two molecules are looked at, but when an entire ensemble of molecules is looked at, behavior acquires meaning. If everyone can be reduced to molecules which obey the same laws of physics, how then are we different from one another? The answer is that we obtain our individuality by what quantities of specific molecules we have, where they are located, and where they are moving to.

Reductionism is neither good nor bad. It either works or it does not in helping us to understand and predict human behavior. We cannot say right now whether it is justified; we will just have to wait and see. However, if it does work, it will profoundly affect how we view ourselves. More than ever, we will have to regard ourselves as molecular machines. There are limits, though, to reductionism, which are part of our fundamental limits to understanding our physical world.

UNCERTAINTY There is a basic uncertainty about atoms and molecules that makes it impossible to understand everything about them and ultimately about ourselves. In principle, if we wished to know everything about our behavior, we would need to know what atoms and molecules we have, precisely the location of them, and the speed with which they were moving to interact with other atoms and molecules. Where they are determines what happens, and when they get there determines how quickly it happens. Unfortunately, the uncertainty principle of physics (formulated by the physicist Warner Heisenberg in 1927) tells us that it is impossible to know *simultaneously* the speed and location of atoms and their electrons with great precision.

The greatest uncertainty is in knowing where the electrons are that orbit around an atom or group of atoms that form a molecule. Electrons determine how a molecule is formed from the various atoms and how it will interact with other atoms and molecules. Thus, knowledge about the location of electrons and where they are going is necessary to make precise predictions of what is going to happen inside our body. If we measure the speed very precisely, there will be great uncertainty in knowing the location of the electron. If we measure its location very precisely, there will be great uncertainty in knowing its speed. It may be quite reasonable to want to know where an atom is located in our brain to within one hundred millionth of an inch in order to predict with great precision the subsequent molecular events that will produce a behavior. The uncertainty that surrounds the accurate prediction of both speed and location at the same time is not due to limitations in our scientific instruments for measuring speed and location, but is part of the nature of the universe as we understand it. No improvements in technology can eliminate this basic uncertainty about ourselves. This uncertainty means we cannot make precise predictions about where atoms and their electrons will be and when they will get there. We may like more order and predictability in our universe, but we do not have it. Even Albert Einstein was troubled by this lack of predictability, as indicated by his famous statement, "God does not play dice." Even Einstein could not stop the dice from rolling and the uncertainty that comes with atoms and molecules.

As atoms become assembled into molecules, and molecules become assembled into cells, and cells into entire organisms, the inherent uncertainty we have been discussing does not disappear, it just becomes very small compared to the uncertainty of our measurements of an entire organism. While we could measure an atom's location to within a hundred millionth of an inch, we could measure a person's location only to within about a hundredth of an inch, because no one can hold his or her body that still. Since we cannot measure the location or speed of a human body that precisely (compared to the location of an atom), then the uncertainty principle does not affect these measurements. Remember that the uncertainty principle comes into play only when we want precise measurements, at the same time, of both location and speed of very very small submicroscopic objects.

We do not know how precisely we would have to determine the speed and location of electrons, atoms, and molecules inside our bodies in order to predict behavior with great accuracy. So the limitations the uncertainty principle presents us with may be of more theoretical than practical importance for now. But there are other problems that limit our understanding of ourselves. Molecules are continually in motion in our bodies (and everywhere else as well), moving to specific locations to perform some function, or just moving about, not going anywhere. In fact, random motion is a property of all molecules in living as well as in nonliving objects; it only ceases to exist at −459°F or −273°C (called absolute zero). Above this temperature, molecules move faster and faster as the temperature increases. Boiling water (212°F), in fact, evaporates because water molecules are moving about so rapidly that they leave the pan. At our body temperature of 98.6°F, molecular motion is less rapid but it is still random, which means we cannot predict where every molecule is going. In spite of molecules moving about at random, things continue to work and we have life. The way cells are structured into tiny compartments insures that eventually enough of the right randomly moving molecules will get to the right places for us to function. The random motion of molecules produces a greater uncertainty in knowing where the molecules are than the uncertainty principle does. The combination of random motion and the uncertainty principle makes it impossible to know what every molecule in our body is going to do. Add to this the obvious fact that there is no way we can make measurements on all our molecules without destroying ourselves. To measure molecules deep within us, we would have to cut away and destroy the molecules of tissue to get at them. If we are looking in the brain, this is a serious limitation. We must conclude that the absolute prediction of behavior (even given the best molecular information) is impossible. Not only is God throwing the dice, but He will not let us look at them. This does not in any way reduce the importance of molecules in our behavior—it merely sets limits on how much we can expect to know about ourselves even when we look for answers at the molecular level. This is where the mystery of life really begins.

ON UNDERSTANDING OUR BRAIN   With such limits, we can well ask the question "Is the human brain capable of understanding itself?" Can we understand ourselves any more than any other machine can? Perhaps we are incapable of understanding ourselves. For example, creative people cannot tell you how they get an idea. All they can say is that an idea occurs to them and then they work out the music, story, theory, design, or whatever around the idea. There may be certain conditions when they think best, such as during sleep, in the morning, during absolute quiet, on a train, etc. But they cannot tell us how their ideas were generated—they do not know. We may be inspired by something we experience, but how the idea pops into our head is the mystery. We have seen that there are sound physical reasons (randomness and the uncertainty principle) for us to doubt that we will obtain a complete understanding of our brain and an understanding of why we do what we do. There may also be other reasons.

The American mathematician Kurt Gödel showed in 1931 that certain observations about mathematics could never be proven (or disproven) within the logical framework of mathematics itself. That is, an observation about numbers could be made that appeared to be true in every respect because no exception to the observation had ever been found. Yet according to Gödel, its truth might never be proven.* Mathematical proofs are not easy to produce.

*For example, the Goldbach conjecture, as it is called, states that all even numbers greater than two are the sum of just two prime numbers. A prime number is a number that is divisible only by one and itself. Thus:

$$
\begin{array}{l}
\text{some} \\
\text{even} \\
\text{numbers}
\end{array}
\left\{
\begin{array}{l}
4 = 3 + 1 \\
6 = 5 + 1 \\
8 = 7 + 1 \quad \text{(Where 1, 3, 5, 7 are prime numbers)} \\
10 = 7 + 3
\end{array}
\right.
$$

If you think about it for a moment, proving $1 + 1 = 2$ is not a simple matter. Why does not $1 + 1 = 11$? You have to define what *1* means, and *2,* and $+$, and $=$, and then we have to agree on the definitions. Gödel is not saying that some mathematical proofs will be difficult. He is saying some proofs will be impossible, not because these mathematical statements we are trying to prove are untrue, but because the logic of mathematics is not powerful enough to prove them. It is like saying that no system can understand itself. To understand one's self, one has to get outside the system (body) and observe. This is physically impossible. Our brain is always between reality and its measurement, as many have pointed out.

A generalization of Gödel's proof (that we cannot prove or disprove everything in mathematics) would be that some observations within any field utilizing logic can never be proven true or false either. Science works within a logical framework of thinking because it depends upon rules for gathering and interpreting data. Science makes generalizations from specific facts that have been discovered (if one bone of a prehistoric animal is found, the size of the entire animal can be determined) and uses generalizations to deal with specific facts (humans have a special skull shape, so finding prehistoric skulls with this shape means that the bones are of human origin). Utilizing logic, science then is subject to the restrictions of logic Gödel

This conjecture is as obviously true for other even numbers as for the ones here, but has not been proven. It may be an example of what Gödel was talking about, but Gödel did not specify how to determine whether something could eventually be proven or not. He only specified that some things cannot be proven.

talks about. Therefore, some scientific statements about the brain can never be proven or disproven, and our knowledge about the brain will always be incomplete. Computers will be no help with this dilemma since they use logic just as we do, and are subject to the same limitations Gödel says exist in any logical system.

It is always fun to show one's superiority to computers, especially when they cannot fight back by sending along another computerized bill. Our brain may have as many as 10^{50} (1 followed by 50 zeros) nerve connections within it. The pathways formed by these connections, you remember from chapter 3, may form the basis of our memory and thinking abilities. To understand fully our abilities may require looking at each connection to see what is there. There are so many connections, however, that even computers could not count all of ours. Let us assume we have a computer one cubic foot in size that can count one connection every billionth of a second (at present there is no computer that can count this fast). If this computer were present and working at the time the earth was formed about five billion years ago, it would now only have counted about 10^{27} connections. If there were one of these computers on every square foot of the earth's surface, piled one hundred miles high (if we are going to speculate, we might as well go all out), it would still have counted only about 10^{49} of the 10^{50} connections! We do have a way to go before a complete understanding of the brain is possible, just in terms of counting the number of brain-cell connections.

This counting limitation, plus Gödel's proof, random molecular motions, and the uncertainty principle set limits to understanding all the molecular and atomic aspects of our behavior. But the study of the molecular basis of behavior is still young, and is a long way from reaching these limits. As of now, there is still far to go before the molecular approach can predict some behaviors as well as you or I can just from experience. We know, for example, that in a crowded theater, the shout of "fire" will drive the people out. We can make this prediction without any knowledge whatever of molecular events in their brains, or in our own, for that matter. There are many other behaviors, however, where simple observation cannot predict what is going to happen or to whom it is going to happen. Some of these behaviors have been the subject of this book.

A REVIEW OF BEHAVIOR   Table 2 lists the behaviors I have discussed in this book and contrasts the traditional or conventional psychological origins of behavior with the more recently formulated biological origins. As I argued in chapter 1, psychological and biological influences on behavior are essentially the same ultimately since both exert their effects through molecular action, but I have used these terms because of their popular meanings. So the issue is not which one has a molecular effect and which one does not. Let me define them more precisely, though. Psychological influences are the effects other people, places, things, and events have upon our behavior. They are what we experience in our surroundings, what we sense of our environment, and what opinions and attitudes we learn from it. Biological influences are those that do not depend upon what we observe around us. These influences do not affect us through our senses, as psycho-

Table 2: ORIGINS OF BEHAVIOR

BEHAVIOR	SOME PSYCHOLOGICAL INFLUENCES	SOME BIOLOGICAL INFLUENCES
*Sexual Desire	Sensory stimulation	Biological clock, hormone levels
*Sleep	Boredom, stress	Biological clock, fever, exercise
Dreaming	Wishes, troubles, memory	Biological clock
Work performance	Sensory stimulation, training	Biological clock
Sensory awareness	Sensory stimulation	Biological clock
Mood	Sensory stimulation	Biological clock
*Intelligence, thinking, decision making	Learning, sensory stimulation	Biological clock, molecular structure of brain, chance
*Creativity	Inspiration from environment	Chance, molecular structure of brain
Motivation	Rewards	Molecular structure of brain
*Certain facial expressions	Learning	Facial muscles and nerves prepro-grammed to control them
Verbal ability	Learning	Molecular structure of female brain
Spatial ability	Learning	Molecular structure of male brain
Impotence	Stress	Testosterone hormone
*Schizophrenia	Stress	Dopamine excess
*Major depression	Stress	Norepinephrine insufficiency
*Anxiety disorder	Fear	Lactic acid excess
*Aggression	Frustration, fear, learning	Molecular structure of brain, hormone levels
Crimes against property	Social conditions, learning	Molecular structure of brain
*Love	Learning	Molecular structure of brain
*Overeating	Sensory stimulation, learning	Metabolism, stomach-chemical signals

*Anorexia nervosa	Disturbed family relationships	Hypothalamus dysfunction
*Alcoholism	Stress	Metabolism
*Homosexuality	Learning, parental influences	Prenatal hormones
Happiness	Sensory stimulation	Brain pleasure center, endorphins
*Temperament	Learning, sensory stimulation	Molecular structure of brain
*Hyperactivity	Inadequate social relations	Food dyes, lead, molecular structure of brain

*Behaviors determined mostly by biological influences; see text.

logical influences do. Things in our environment that might affect our behavior in a biological way—such as diseases, infections, or poor nutrition—enter our body without any initial sensory awareness on our part. We do not know when bacteria enter our body; we only know this after the bacteria cause a problem. We are not aware at the time of eating that we are not getting enough vitamins; we only know this after a vitamin-deficiency disease develops. Other biological influences originate within the body and depend upon genetic, physiological, and random influences. In short, what information we take in through our five senses is psychological, and everything else is biological.

Both the psychological and biological influences play a part in the origin of all our behaviors, but not necessarily equal parts. I have indicated with an asterisk in Table 2 those behaviors I think depend most on biological influences and hence the least on psychological influences. Each of these behaviors was, of course, discussed in the preceding chapters. To put it simply, all behaviors depend mostly on biological influences, because without the biology we would not have a body to begin with. But given a body and all the genes to direct its assembly, and the nutrients to make it grow and maintain itself, then one can ask what relative contribution psychological influences have. Most people think they know anyhow. If they are a success it is because of biological influences (guts, hard work, brains). If they are failures, it is because of the environment (people or events did them in).

WHAT SHOULD WE DO?   Given what we know and what we might know about behavior, is there any message to us about how we should behave? The usual conclusion is that science can tell us what *is*, but not what *ought to be*. That is, science gathers facts but cannot tell us how to use these facts. Science can put its facts together to build an atomic weapon, but these facts do not tell us whether we ought to use it. Similarly, science can find the cause of homosexuality and give us the facts to change it, but these facts alone cannot tell us whether we ought to change it. What ought to be is considered a matter of policy—a matter of judgment and an opinion based on what facts a policymaker wishes to use.

How we ought to behave, then, is a matter of values. Is it good to marry and not have children; is it bad to fight others; should we reduce the obese, convert nonbelievers, or ban abortions? We all have opinions about what we ought to do, but they are not formulated outside of the body, they are formulated in the brain. If it is in the brain, it is subject to study, so values have a biological basis. In order to formulate our values we need some facts in our memory. The facts may be what we have been taught or what we have learned ourselves. Then in order to formulate values, we need decision making within our brains to choose among alternative courses of action. Some people would require vast amounts of information before they could formulate any values. Others would need only minimal information. They hear it, they believe it and that's that. Value development depends, therefore, on what is in memory as facts and on how the decision-making processes of the brain deal with these facts to create an opinion. So in the brain, what *is* determines what *ought to be*. As we learn more about brain function, this should all become a lot clearer. We can say now, however, that because of differences among people in how their memory and decision-making processes operate, no one value will emerge that we can all agree on. There will be majority opinions but not unanimous ones. Given exactly the same facts, different opinions of what we should do will always emerge. Opinion polls never show complete agreement among people where values are concerned. We need not even go this far, as friends and family seldom agree on everything either.

What we ought to do, how we ought to behave, is determined by the brain and not by science. So our initial statement remains intact: Science cannot tell us what ought to be. Science will be able to tell us how our brain does it, but since every brain does it differently, there is no way to determine who does it best. Therefore there is no way to tell us which values are best. In addition, what ought to be often depends not only on one person's judgment, but also on what others think. What the United

States thinks it ought to do in its foreign relations may not be what other countries think it ought to do. How you wish to live your life may not agree with how others think you should live it.

SOME CAUTIONS   From reading this book, some cautions in dealing with behavior should be apparent. In view of the molecular nature of all behaviors, beware of theories of behavior that are exclusively psychological (as defined for Table 2) and that ignore the biological components. All behaviors have to have a biological basis upon which the psychological influences are laid down. To propose only a psychological theory of behavior is to be incomplete. In view of what it takes to prove a psychological cause of behavior, beware of studies that claim to prove how a behavior developed. A shared opinion among a group of professionals about the cause of a behavior does not constitute scientific proof. Well-controlled studies have to be conducted and alternative explanations ruled out. Adoption studies of identical twins are the closest we can come to establishing proof for the psychological causes of behavior. In view of the uncertainty in studying matter, beware of any reported complete explanation of behavior, as there can never be one. We cannot know what all molecules in the body are doing at any given time. Consequently, a totally accurate prediction of what any given individual will do in any given situation will not be possible. People are the most complex things in the world.

A MOLECULAR TOMORROW   As the molecules that control our behavior become identified, and as we understand their interaction with other molecules in our body, we will begin to achieve power over the human species in a way we have never had before. We will confront life on its own level, molecule for molecule. This knowledge will change the way we look at ourselves. It will cause problems for us because everything we create, including more people, causes us problems. One problem it is going to create is whether we tell people after we have analyzed their molecules what behaviors they are likely to exhibit. Does telling them resign them to do what we predict they are likely to do (a self-fulfilling prophecy) or does it give them guidelines to live within? If we tell certain people that they have the enzymes likely to make them obese or alcoholic, they can watch their food and alcoholic intake more carefully. On the other hand, if we tell certain people they are likely to become schizophrenic or severely depressed, then they are going to worry about it and disrupt their lives.

When we try to influence other people, we are in effect trying to change their brain chemistry. Our parents try to influence us, as do our friends, teachers, salespeople, advertisers, politicans, preachers, and all sorts of organizations. This is all perfectly legal, moral, and nonfattening, as long as they do not physically touch us. Just as they are free to try and influence us, we are free not to be influenced if we do not wish to be. It is a game, in a sense.

There is another game played where behavior is not changed but is selected from the available pool of people. The game is genetically based, but it is not called that. Military aircraft pilots are selected for training on the basis of their eye-hand coordination, depth perception, and general vision. Basketball players are selected for their height and fast reflexes. Crews for ocean racing yachts are not selected if they have inner ear problems and get seasick. Some music teachers do not put youngsters on brass instruments if they do not have the right facial and tongue muscles to make a sound pretty quickly through the mouthpiece. High-fashion models in the United States are selected on the basis of having high cheekbones, long necks, and a modest bust. All these selection criteria are essentially genetic in nature (genes are involved in producing what is selected), but nobody complains. We have been making genetically based decisions for a long time. But soon it will be tempting, with our molecular knowledge, to change physically the things we do not like and to amplify the things we do like, and not just select for certain genes. Block a molecule here, speed up another there. Get them by their molecules and their hearts and minds will follow. When we see what may be possible and how much we can change ourselves by tampering with our molecules with genetic engineering, with pills, injections, or whatever, we may decide that we will work harder with the social, psychological, and environmental tools that we have in order to avoid biological intervention and its consequences. We will have the power to change ourselves beyond recognition. If the recognition is lost, let us hope it is because we have never looked better, and not because we have become too horrible to contemplate.

Books and Articles That Helped in Writing This Book

Chapter 1. Molecular Gods at Work

Beck, William S. *Human Design.* New York: Harcourt Brace Jovanovich, 1971.

Boddy, John. *Brain Systems and Psychological Concepts.* New York: Wiley, 1978.

Bracewell, Ronald N. *The Galactic Club—Intelligent Life in Outer Space.* San Francisco: W. H. Freeman, 1974.

Caplan, David, ed. *Biological Studies of Mental Processes.* Cambridge: M.I.T. Press, 1980.

De Cayeux, André. *Three Billion Years of Life.* New York: Stein and Day, 1970.

D'Espagnat, Bernard. "The Quantum Theory and Reality." *Scientific American,* Nov. 1979, p. 158.

Guyton, Arthur C. *Structure and Function of the Nervous System.* Philadelphia: W. B. Saunders, 1972.

Jastrow, Robert. *God and the Astronomers.* New York: W. W. Norton, 1978.

Kaplan, Abraham. *The Conduct of Inquiry.* San Francisco: Chandler Publishing Co., 1964.

Koestler, Arthur. *The Ghost in the Machine.* Chicago: Henry Regnery Co., 1967.

Miller, James G. *Living Systems.* New York: McGraw-Hill, 1978.

Monod, Jacques. *Chance and Necessity.* New York: Vintage Books, 1972.

Schrödinger, Erwin. *What Is Life?* New York: Doubleday, 1956.

Uttal, William R. *The Psychobiology of Sensory Coding.* New York: Harper and Row, 1973.

White, Abraham, et al. *Principles of Biochemistry,* 6th ed. New York: McGraw-Hill, 1978.

Zander, Alvin. "The Psychology of Group Processes." *Annual Review of Psychology,* Vol. 30 (1979), p. 417.

*Chapter 2.*Biological Rhythms

Allison, Truett, and Domenic V. Cicchetti. "Sleep in Mammals: Ecological and Constitutional Correlates." *Science,* Vol. 194 (1976), p. 732.

Armitage, Sally E., et al. "The Fetal Sound Environment of Sheep." *Science,* Vol. 208 (1980), p. 1173.

Bünning, Erwin. *The Physiological Clock,* 3rd ed. New York: Springer-Verlag, 1973.

Cartwright, Rosalind D. *A Primer on Sleep and Dreaming.* Reading, Mass.: Addison-Wesley, 1978.

Comfort, Alex. *The Biology of Senescence.* New York: Elsevier, 1979.

Doob, Leonard W. *Patterning of Time.* New Haven: Yale University Press, 1971.

Ehret, Charles F., et al. "Chronotypic Action of Theophylline and of Pentobarbital as Circadian Zeitgebers in the Rat." *Science,* Vol. 188 (1975), p. 1212.

Freemon, Frank R. *Sleep Research.* Springfield, Ill.: Charles C. Thomas, 1972.

Hayflick, Leonard. "The Cell Biology of Human Aging." *Scientific American,* Jan. 1980, p. 58.

Holmes, David S., et al. "Biorhythms: Their Utility for Predicting Postoperative Recuperative Time, Death, and Athletic Performance." *Journal of Applied Psychology,* Vol. 65 (1980), p. 233.

Jacobs, Barry L., and Michael E. Trulson. "Dreams, Hallucinations, and Psychosis—The Serotonin Connection." *Trends in Neurosciences,* Nov. 1979, p. 276.

Klein, K. E., et al. "Air Operations and Circadian Performance Rhythms." *Aviation Space and Environmental Medicine,* Vol. 47 (1976), p. 221.

Luce, Gay G. *Biological Rhythms in Human and Animal Physiology.* New York: Dover, 1971.

Palmer, John D. *An Introduction to Biological Rhythms.* New York: Academic Press, 1976.

Pappenheimer, John R. "The Sleep Factor." *Scientific American,* Aug. 1976, p. 24.

Sugarman, Gerald I., et al. "Cockayne Syndrome: Clinical Study of

Two Patients and Neuropathological Findings in One." *Clinical Pediatrics,* Vol. 16 (1977), p. 225.

Sulloway, Frank J. *Freud, Biologist of the Mind.* New York: Basic Books, 1979.

Timiras, Paola S. "Biological Perspectives on Aging." *American Scientist,* Sept.–Oct. 1978, p. 605.

Ward, Ritchie R. *The Living Clocks.* New York: Mentor, 1971.

Wehr, Thomas A., et al. "Phase Advance of the Circadian Sleep-Wake Cycle as an Antidepressant." *Science,* Vol. 206 (1979), p. 710.

Weston, Lee. *Body Rhythm.* New York: Harcourt Brace Jovanovich, 1979.

Wolman, Benjamin B., ed. *Handbook of Dreams.* New York: Van Nostrand Reinhold, 1979.

Zimbardo, Philip G., et al. "Objective Assessment of Hypnotically Induced Time Distortion." *Science,* Vol. 181 (1973), p. 282.

*Chapter 3.*Thinking

Altman, Joseph. *Organic Foundations of Animal Behavior.* New York: Holt Rinehart and Winston, 1966.

Arnold, Arthur P. "Sexual Differences in the Brain." *American Scientist,* Mar.–Apr. 1980, p. 165.

Bartus, Raymond T. "Physostigmine and Recent Memory: Effects in Young and Aged Nonhuman Primates." *Science,* Vol. 206 (1979), p. 1087.

———, et al. "Age-Related Changes in Passive Avoidance Retention: Modulation With Dietary Choline." *Science,* Vol. 209 (1980), p. 301.

Blakemore, Colin. *Mechanics of the Mind.* Cambridge: Cambridge University Press, 1977.

"The Brain." *Scientific American,* Sept. 1979. Entire issue.

Buell, Stephen J., and Paul D. Coleman. "Dendritic Growth in the Aged Human Brain and Failure of Growth in Senile Dementia." *Science,* Vol. 206 (1979), p. 854.

Bullock, Theodore H. *Introduction to Nervous Systems.* San Francisco: W. H. Freeman, 1977.

Dennett, Daniel C. *Brainstorms: Philosophical Essays on Mind and Psychology.* Montgomery, Vt.: Bradford Books, 1978.

Diamond, Marian C. "The Aging Brain: Some Enlightening and Optimistic Results." *American Scientist,* Jan.–Feb. 1978, p. 66.

Dunn, Adrian J. "Neurochemistry of Learning and Memory: An Evaluation of Recent Data." *Annual Review of Psychology*, Vol. 31 (1980), p. 343.

Eccles, John C. *The Understanding of the Brain*, 2nd ed. New York: McGraw-Hill, 1977.

Eibl-Eibesfeldt, Irenäus. *Ethology*, 2nd ed. New York: Holt Rinehart and Winston, 1975.

Ekman, Paul, and Harriet Oster. "Facial Expressions of Emotion." *Annual Review of Psychology*, Vol. 30 (1979), p. 527.

Galaburda, Albert M., et al. "Right-Left Asymmetries in the Brain." *Science*, Vol. 199 (1978), p. 852.

Gazzaniga, Michael S., and Joseph E. LeDoux. *The Integrated Mind*. New York: Plenum Press, 1978.

Gillam, Barbara. "Geometrical Illusions." *Scientific American*, Jan. 1980, p. 102.

Hartmann, Ernest L. *The Functions of Sleep*. New Haven: Yale University Press, 1973,

Jaynes, Julian. *The Origin of Consciousness in the Breakdown of the Bicameral Mind*. Boston: Houghton-Mifflin, 1976.

Kolata, Gina Bari. "Sex Hormones and Brain Development." *Science*, Vol. 205 (1979), p. 985.

Lassen, Niels A., et al. "Brain Function and Blood Flow." *Scientific American*, Oct. 1978, p. 62.

Maccoby, Eleanor E., and Carol N. Jacklin. *The Psychology of Sex Differences*. Stanford, Calif.: Stanford University Press, 1974.

Mason, Stephen T. "Noradrenaline and Behaviour." *Trends in Neurosciences*, Mar. 1979, p. 82.

Mc Glone, Jeannette, et al. "Six Differences in Human Brain Asymmetry: A Critical Survey." *The Behavioral and Brain Sciences*, Vol. 3 (1980), p. 215.

Ornstein, Robert E. *On the Experience of Time*. Baltimore: Penguin Books, 1970.

Reed, Graham. *The Psychology of Anomalous Experience*. Boston: Houghton-Mifflin, 1972.

Regan, David. "Electrical Responses Evoked From the Human Brain." *Scientific American*, Dec. 1979, p. 134.

Restak, Richard M. *The Brain*. New York: Doubleday, 1979.

Rose, Steven. *The Conscious Brain*. New York: Vintage Books, 1976.

Rovet, J., and C. Netley. "Phenotypic vs. Genotypic Sex and Cognitive Abilities." *Behavior Genetics*, Vol. 9 (1979), p. 317.

Stellar, Eliot, and John D. Corbit, eds. "Neural Control of Motivated Behavior." *Neurosciences Research Program Bulletin*, Vol. 11, No. 4 (1973).

Books and Articles That Helped In Writing This Book

Yesavage, Jerome. "Memory, Lost and Found." *The Stanford Magazine,* Spring–Summer 1980, p. 36.

Young, J. Z. *Programs of the Brain.* Oxford: Oxford University Press, 1978.

Chapter 4. Molecular Psychiatry

Bacopoulos, N. C., et al. "Antipsychotic Drug Action in Schizophrenic Patients: Effect on Cortical Dopamine Metabolism After Long-Term Treatment." *Science,* Vol. 205 (1979), p. 1405.

Barchas, Jack D., et al. "Behavioral Neurochemistry: Neuroregulators and Behavioral States." *Science,* Vol. 200 (1978), p. 964.

Berger, Philip A. "Medical Treatment of Mental Illness." *Science,* Vol. 200 (1978), p. 974.

Bird, Edward D., et al. "Brain Norepinephrine and Dopamine in Schizophrenia." *Science,* Vol. 204 (1979), p. 93.

Bloom, Floyd, et al. "Endorphins: Profound Behavioral Effects in Rats Suggest New Etiological Factors in Mental Illness." *Science,* Vol. 194 (1976), p. 630.

Brooks, Benjamin R., et al. "Slow Viral Infections." *Annual Review of Neuroscience,* Vol. 2 (1979), p. 309.

DeWied, D. "Schizophrenia as an Inborn Error in the Degradation of Beta-Endorphin—A Hypothesis." *Trends in Neurosciences,* Mar. 1979, p. 79.

Diagnostic and Statistical Manual of Mental Disorders, 3rd ed. American Psychiatric Association, Washington, D. C., 1980.

Fieve, Ronald R., et al., eds. *Genetic Research in Psychiatry.* Baltimore: Johns Hopkins University Press, 1975.

Frazer, Alan, and Andrew Winokur, eds. *Biological Bases of Psychiatric Disorders.* New York: Spectrum Publications, 1977.

Gross, Martin L. *The Psychological Society.* New York: Random House, 1978.

Heston, Leonard L. "The Genetics of Schizophrenia and Schizoid Disease." *Science,* Vol. 167 (1970), p. 249.

Hirsch, Steven R. "Do Parents Cause Schizophrenia?" *Trends in Neurosciences,* Feb. 1979, p. 49.

Horrobin, David. "A Singular Solution for Schizophrenia." *New Scientist,* Vol. 85 (1980), p. 642.

Kolata, Gina Bari. "Mental Disorders: A New Approach to Treatment?" *Science,* Vol. 203 (1979), p. 36.

Lake, C. R., et al. "Schizophrenia: Elevated Cerebrospinal Fluid Norepinephrine." *Science,* Vol. 207 (1980), p. 331.

Marshall, Eliot. "Psychotherapy Works, But for Whom?" *Science,* Vol. 207 (1980), p. 506.

Murphy, Jane M. "Psychiatric Labeling in Cross-Cultural Perspective." *Science,* Vol. 191 (1976), p. 1019.

Nicholi, Armand M., Jr., ed. *The Harvard Guide to Modern Psychiatry.* Cambridge: Harvard University Press, 1978.

Pauling, Linus. "Orthomolecular Psychiatry." *Science,* Vol. 160 (1968), p. 265.

Pincus, Jonathan H., and Gary J. Tucker. *Behavioral Neurology,* 2nd ed. New York: Oxford University Press, 1978.

Pitts, Ferris N., Jr. "Biochemical Factors in Anxiety Neurosis." *Behavioral Science,* Vol. 16 (1971), p. 82.

Rosenhan, D. L. "On Being Sane in Insane Places." *Science,* Vol. 179 (1973), p. 250.

Rosenthal, David. *Genetics of Psychopathology.* New York: McGraw-Hill, 1971.

Ross, Maureen, et al. "Plasma Beta-Endorphin Immunoreactivity in Schizophrenia." *Science,* Vol. 205 (1979), p. 1163.

Sachar, Edward J., and Miron Baron. "The Biology of Affective Disorders." *Annual Review of Neuroscience,* Vol. 2 (1979), p. 505.

Schulsinger, Fini. "Biological Psychopathology." *Annual Review of Psychology,* Vol. 31 (1980), p. 583.

Snyder, Solomon H., and Steven R. Childers. "Opiate Receptors and Opioid Peptides." *Annual Review of Neurosciences,* Vol. 2 (1979), p. 35.

Spark, Richard F., et al. "Impotence Is Not Always Psychogenic." *The Journal of the American Medical Association,* Vol. 243 (1980), p. 750.

Tallman, John F., et al. "Receptors for the Age of Anxiety: Pharmacology of the Benzodiazepines." *Science,* Vol. 207 (1980), p. 274.

Trulson, Michael E., and Barry L. Jacobs. "Long-Term Amphetamine Treatment Decreases Brain Serotonin Metabolism: Implications for Theories of Schizophrenia." *Science,* Vol. 205 (1979), p. 1295.

Worden, Frederic G., et al., eds. "Frontiers of Psychiatric Genetics." *Neurosciences Research Program Bulletin,* Vol. 14, No. 1 (1976).

*Chapter 5.*Love and Hate

Barash, David. *The Whisperings Within.* New York: Harper and Row, 1979.

Books and Articles That Helped In Writing This Book

Berkowitz, Leonard. "Simple Views of Aggression." *American Scientist,* Vol. 57 (1969), p. 372.

Bronson, F. H., and Claude Desjardins. "Aggression in Adult Mice: Modification by Neonatal Injections of Gonadal Hormones." *Science,* Vol. 161 (1968), p. 705.

Colinvaux, Paul. *Why Big Fierce Animals Are Rare.* Princeton: Princeton University Press, 1978.

Datesman, Susan K., and Frank R. Scarpitti, eds. *Women, Crime, and Justice.* New York: Oxford University Press, 1980.

Delgado, José M. R. *Physical Control of the Mind.* New York: Harper and Row, 1969.

Edwards, David A. "Mice: Fighting by Neonatally Androgenized Females." *Science,* Vol. 161 (1968), p. 1027.

Freedman, Daniel G. *Human Sociobiology.* New York: Free Press, 1979.

Fromm, Erich. *The Anatomy of Human Destructiveness.* New York: Holt Rinehart and Winston, 1973.

Hinde, Robert A. *Biological Bases of Human Social Behavior.* New York: McGraw-Hill, 1974.

Holden, Constance. "The Criminal Mind: A New Look at an Ancient Puzzle." *Science,* Vol. 199 (1978), p. 511.

Leakey, Richard E., and Roger Lewin. *Origins.* New York: E. P. Dutton, 1977.

Lewis, Dorothy O., et al. "Violent Juvenile Delinquents: Psychiatric, Neurological, Psychological and Abuse Factors." *Journal of the American Academy of Child Psychiatry,* Vol. 18 (1979), p. 307.

Lunde, Donald T. *Murder and Madness.* San Francisco: San Francisco Book Co., 1976.

Mark, Vernon H., and Frank R. Ervin. *Violence and the Brain.* New York: Harper and Row, 1970.

McCord, Joan. "Some Child Rearing Antecedents of Criminal Behavior in Adult Men." *Journal of Personality and Social Psychology,* Vol. 37 (1979), p. 1477.

Mednick, Sarnoff A., and Karl O. Christiansen, eds. *Biosocial Bases of Criminal Behavior.* New York: Gardner Press, 1977.

Money, John. *Love and Lovesickness.* Baltimore: Johns Hopkins University Press, 1980.

Montagu, Ashley. *The Nature of Human Aggression.* New York: Oxford University Press, 1976.

Roche, Kerry E., and Alan I. Leshner. "ACTH and Vasopressin Treatments Immediately After a Defeat Increase Future Submissiveness in Male Mice." *Science,* Vol. 204 (1979), p. 1343.

Ruse, Michael. *Sociobiology: Sense or Nonsense?* Boston: D. Reidel
   Publishing Co., 1979.
Scott, John Paul. *Aggression,* 2nd ed. Chicago: University of Chicago
   Press, 1975.
Silberman, Charles E. *Criminal Violence, Criminal Justice.* New York:
   Random House, 1978.
Smith, Douglas E., et al. "Lateral Hypothalamic Control of Killing:
   Evidence for a Cholinoceptive Mechanism." *Science,* Vol. 167
   (1970), p. 900.
Tinbergen, N. "On War and Peace in Animals and Man." *Science,*
   Vol. 160 (1968), p. 1411.
Vernon, Walter, "Animal Aggression: Review of Research." *Genetic
   Psychology Monographs,* Vol. 80 (1969), p. 3.
Vom Saal, Frederick S., et al. "Time of Neonatal Androgen Exposure
   Influences Length of Testosterone Treatment Required to
   Induce Aggression in Adult Male and Female Mice." *Behavioral
   Biology,* Vol. 17 (1976), p. 391.
Wallace, Robert A. *The Genesis Factor.* New York: William Morrow,
   1979.
Washburn, Sherwood. "The Evolution of Man." *Scientific American,*
   Sept. 1978, p. 194.
Witkin, Herman A., et al. "Criminality in XYY and XXY Men."
   Science, Vol. 193 (1976), p. 547.

*Chapter 6.*Molecular Self-Improvement

Ahlskog, J. Eric, and Bartley G. Hoebel. "Overeating and Obesity
   From Damage to a Noradrenergic System in the Brain." *Science,*
   Vol. 182 (1973), p. 166.
Augustine, George J., Jr., and Herbert Levitan. "Neurotransmitter
   Release From a Vertebrate Neuromuscular Synapse Affected by
   a Food Dye." *Science,* Vol. 207 (1980), p. 1489.
Bemis, Kelly M. "Current Approaches to the Etiology and Treatment
   of Anorexia Nervosa." *Psychological Bulletin,* Vol. 85 (1978),
   p. 593.
Berkow, Robert, et al., eds. *The Merck Manual of Diagnosis and
   Therapy,* 13th ed. Rahway, N. J.: Merck, Sharp and Dohme
   Research Laboratories, 1977.
Bermant, Gordon, and Julian M. Davidson. *Biological Bases of Sexual
   Behavior.* New York: Harper and Row, 1974.

Books and Articles That Helped In Writing This Book

Betz, Barbara J., and Caroline B. Thomas. "Individual Temperament as a Predictor of Health or Pre-Mature Disease." *Johns Hopkins Medical Journal,* Vol. 144 (1979), p. 81.

Boddy, John. *Brain Systems and Psychological Concepts.* New York: Wiley, 1978.

Bruch, Hilde. *Eating Disorders.* New York: Basic Books, 1973.

Carey, Gregory, et al. "Genetics and Personality Inventories: The Limits of Replication With Twin Data." *Behavior Genetics,* Vol. 8 (1978), p. 299.

Coleman, Douglas L. "Obesity Genes: Beneficial Effects in Heterozygous Mice." *Science,* Vol. 203 (1979), p. 663.

Cox, Tom, *Stress.* Baltimore: University Park Press, 1978.

Della-Fera, Mary Ann, and Clifton A. Baile. "Cholecystokinin Octapeptide: Continuous Picomole Injections Into the Cerebral Ventricles of Sheep Suppress Feeding." *Science,* Vol. 206 (1979), p. 471.

Dobzhansky, Theodosius. *The Biological Basis of Human Freedom.* New York: Columbia University Press, 1956.

Dworkin, Robert H., et al. "A Longitudinal Study of the Genetics of Personality." *Journal of Personality and Social Psychology,* Vol. 34 (1976), p. 510.

Ehrhardt, Anke A., and Heino F. L. Meyer-Bahlburg. "Prenatal Sex Hormones and the Developing Brain." *Annual Review of Medicine,* Vol. 30 (1979), p. 417.

Epstein, Seymour. "The Stability of Behavior: I. On Predicting Most of the People Much of the Time." *Journal of Personality and Social Psychology,* Vol. 37 (1979), p. 1097.

Eriksson, C. J. Peter, and Marc A. Schuckit. "Elevated Blood Acetaldehyde Levels in Alchoholics and Their Relatives: A Reevaluation." *Science,* Vol. 207 (1980), p. 1383.

Freed, William J., et al. "Calcitonin: Inhibitory Effect on Eating in Rats." *Science,* Vol. 206 (1979), p. 850.

Fuller, John L. *Foundations of Behavior Genetics.* St. Louis: Mosby, 1978.

Holden, Constance. "Identical Twins Reared Apart." *Science,* Vol. 207 (1980), p. 1323.

———. "Rand Issues Final Alcoholism Report." *Science,* Vol. 207 (1980), p. 855.

Karlsson, Jon L. *Inheritance of Creative Intelligence.* Chicago: Nelson-Hall, 1978.

Kolata, Gina Bari. "Obesity." *Science,* Vol. 198 (1977), p. 905.

Leshner, Alan I. *An Introduction to Behavioral Endocrinology.* New York: Oxford University Press, 1978.

Lieber, Charles S. "The Metabolism of Alcohol." *Scientific American,*
  Mar. 1976, p. 25.

Loraine, J. A., ed. *Understanding Homosexuality: Its Biological and
  Psychological Bases.* New York: American Elsevier, 1974.

Margules, David L., et al. "Beta-Endorphin Is Associated With
  Overeating in Genetically Obese Mice and Rats." *Science,* Vol. 202
  (1978), p. 988.

Marx, Jean L. "Stress." *Science,* Vol. 198 (1977), p. 905.

Masters, W. H., and V. Johnson. *Homosexuality in Perspective.* Boston:
  Little, Brown, 1979.

Mitchell, Terence R. "Organizational Behavior." *Annual Review of
  Psychology,* Vol. 30 (1979), p. 243.

Money, John, and Anke A. Ehrhardt. *Man and Woman, Boy and Girl.*
  New York: Mentor, 1972.

Pihl, R. O., and M. Parkes. "Hair Element Content in Learning
  Disabled Children." *Science,* Vol. 198 (1977), p. 204.

Rabkin, Judith G., and Elmer L. Struening. "Life Events, Stress, and
  Illness." *Science,* Vol. 194 (1976), p. 1013.

Reynolds, Vernon. *The Biology of Human Action.* San Francisco: W. H.
  Freeman, 1976.

Routtenberg, Aryeh. "The Reward System of the Brain." *Scientific
  American,* Nov. 1978, p. 154.

Sahlins, Marshall. *The Use and Abuse of Biology.* Ann Arbor: University
  of Michigan Press, 1976.

Schaie, K. Warner, and Iris A. Parham. "Stability of Adult
  Personality Traits: Fact or Fable?" *Journal of Personality and Social
  Psychology,* Vol. 34 (1976), p. 146.

Schuckit, Marc A., and Vidamantas Rayses. "Ethanol Ingestion:
  Differences in Blood Acetaldehyde Concentrations in Relatives of
  Alcoholics and Controls." *Science,* Vol. 203 (1979), p. 54.

Seixas, Frank A., et al., eds. "Medical Consequences of Alcoholism,"
  Annals of the New York Academy of Sciences, Vol. 252 (1975).

Selye, Hans. "The Evolution of the Stress Concept." *American Scientist,*
  Nov.–Dec. 1973, p. 692.

————. *The Stress of Life,* rev. ed. New York: McGraw-Hill, 1976.

Sex, Hormones and Behavior. Ciba Foundation Symposium 62.
  Amsterdam: Excerpta Medica, 1979.

Shapiro, Bernard H., et al. "The Testicular Feminized Rat: A
  Naturally Occurring Model of Androgen Independent Brain
  Masculinization." *Science,* Vol. 209 (1980), p. 418.

Straus, Eugene, and Rosalyn S. Yalow. "Cholecystokinin in the Brains
  of Obese and Nonobese Mice." *Science,* Vol. 203 (1979), p. 68.

Swanson, James M., and Marcel Kinsbourne. "Food Dyes Impair

Performance of Hyperactive Children on a Laboratory Learning Task." *Science*, Vol. 207 (1980), p. 1485.

Thomas, Alexander, et al. "The Origin of Personality." *Scientific American*, Aug. 1970, p. 102.

Waldrop, Mary F., et al. "Newborn Minor Physical Anomalies Predict Short Attention Span, Peer Aggression, and Impulsivity at Age 3." *Science*, Vol. 199 (1978), p. 563.

Ward, Ingeborg L. "Prenatal Stress Feminizes and Demasculinizes the Behavior of Males." *Science*, Vol. 175 (1972), p. 82.

Ward, Ingeborg L., and Judith Weisz. "Maternal Stress Alters Plasma Testosterone in Fetal Males." *Science*, Vol. 207 (1980), p. 328.

Weiss, Bernard, et al. "Behavioral Responses to Artificial Food Colors." *Science*, Vol. 207 (1980), p. 1487.

Weiss, Gabrielle, and Lily Hechtman. "The Hyperactive Child Syndrome." *Science*, Vol. 205 (1979), p. 1348.

Wolff, Peter H., and Richard Ferber. "The Development of Behavior in Human Infants, Premature and Newborn." *Annual Review of Neuroscience*, Vol. 2 (1979), p. 291.

Wurtman, Judith J., and Richard J. Wurtman. "Sucrose Consumption Early in Life Fails to Modify the Appetite of Adult Rats for Sweet Foods." *Science*, Vol. 205 (1979), p. 321.

*Chapter 7.*Molecular Bondage

Baker, Adolph. *Modern Physics and Antiphysics*. Reading, Mass.: Addison-Wesley, 1970.

Burgers, J. M. "Causality and Anticipation." *Science*, Vol. 189 (1975), p. 194.

The Centrality of Science and Absolute Values, Vol. 1. Proceedings of the Fourth International Conference on the Unity of the Sciences, 1975. The International Cultural Foundation, Tarrytown, N.Y.

Emery, Alan E. H. *Elements of Medical Genetics*, 5th ed. Edinburgh: Churchill Livingstone, 1979.

"Evolution." *Scientific American*, Sept. 1978. Entire issue.

Gould, Stephen Jay. *Ever Since Darwin*. New York: W. W. Norton, 1977.

Harris, Marvin. *Cannibals and Kings*. New York: Random House, 1977.

Hofstadter, Douglas R. *Gödel, Escher, Bach*. New York: Basic Books, 1979.

Lappé, Marc. *Genetic Politics*. New York: Simon and Schuster, 1979.

Books and Articles That Helped In Writing This Book

Matisoo, Juri. "The Superconducting Computer." *Scientific American*, May 1980, p. 50.

Moore, Andrew M. T. "A Pre-Neolithic Farmer's Village on the Euphrates." *Scientific American*, Aug. 1979, p. 62.

Nagel, Ernest, and James R. Newman. "Gödel's Proof," *The World of Mathematics*, Vol. 3. James R. Newman, ed. New York: Simon and Schuster, 1956.

Skinner, B. F. *Beyond Freedom and Dignity*. New York: Alfred A. Knopf, 1971.

Smullyan, Raymond. *What Is the Name of This Book?* Englewood Cliffs, N. J.: Prentice-Hall, 1978.

Thorpe, W. H. *Purpose in a World of Chance*. Oxford: Oxford University Press, 1978.

Weisskopf, Victor F. "The Frontiers and Limits of Science." *American Scientist*, July–Aug. 1977, p. 405.

Wilson, Edward O. *On Human Nature*. Cambridge: Harvard University Press, 1978.

Zukav, Gary. *The Dancing Wu Li Masters*. New York: Morrow, 1979.

Many of these references were useful beyond just the chapters indicated.

Index

Index

Index